CONTENTS

KETO DIET FOR BEGINNERS

INTERMITTENT FASTING

KETO DIET FOR BEGINNERS

Easy Everyday Low Carb Recipes

15-Day Meal Plan

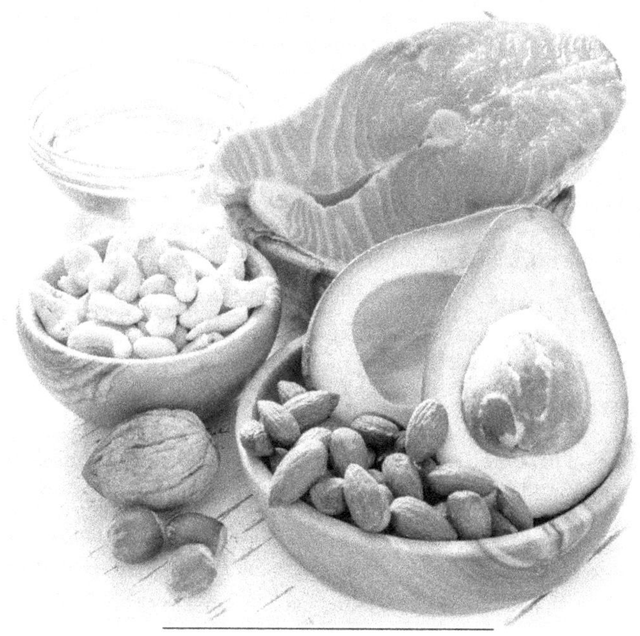

Kierra Lewis

INTRODUCTION

Congratulations on purchasing the *Keto Diet for Beginners: Easy Everyday Low Carb Recipes – 15-Day Meal Plan* and thank you for doing so. The following chapters will discuss how to achieve weight loss, and what you'll need to do to reduce your carbohydrate intake and achieve ketosis. The Keto plan will help you feel full and satisfied while still losing weight. You merely restrict carb intake including starches such as bread and pasta as well as sugars. As a result of the keto diet, you will replace the unwanted elements with fat and protein.

Not only will you lose weight, but you will also lower your triglycerides, blood pressure, and blood sugar. There is no set rule for carb intake. These are some of the basic guidelines to consider as you blaze the path on the ketogenic diet plan:

- 20-50 *Grams Each Day:* If you have diabetes, are obese, or metabolically deranged, this is the plan for you. If you are consuming less than the 50 grams daily; your body will achieve a ketosis state which supplies the ketone bodies.

- *100-150 Grams Each Day*: Stay within these limits if you are active and lean trying to maintain weight.

As you now see, it is important to experiment and categorize where you fall on the scales before you make any changes. As with any new diet changes, you should seek your doctor's advice.

HOW THE KETOGENIC DIET WORKS

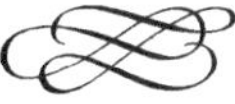

The route you choose will involve flexibility. Depending on your situation, you may not have the same goals as another person. These three categories are the possible levels for you to choose from before you begin. For now, as a beginner, you will be using the first method.

P*lan # 1*: The standard ketogenic diet (SKD) consists of moderate protein, high-fat, and is low in carbs. If you choose to use the SKD dietary approach, you will probably be taking in an average of 30 grams or fewer carbs daily. This will allow you to stay in ketosis which is one of the primary purposes for restriction of your carbohydrates.

P*lan # 2*: The targeted keto diet (TKD) will provide you with the nutrients needed during workout times or at other times when you're more active. The primary goal of the

TKD method is to maintain muscle glycogen and blood sugar at a moderate level for training. You may discover you need to advance to the TKD diet if you are using the SDK plan for approximately 5 weeks. You should begin by introducing 20 to 30 fast-acting carbs approximately 30 minutes prior to your workout time. That should help you when you lift weights on a non-competitive level.

P*lan* # 3: The cyclical ketogenic diet (CKD) is a unique method used with a restrictive 5-day keto diet plan during the times of the day when you're more active. Bodybuilders and athletes are prime examples of people that would be using the CKD method. They have a high-volume and intensity which is needed for trying to optimize their performance. They cannot train properly without the help of carbohydrates. For that reason, it is very important for them to implement the carbohydrate refeeding days one to two times a week to help keep the glycogen in storage at an adequate amount of sugar to fuel their training workouts.

P*lan* # 4: The high-protein keto diet (HPKD) is comparable to the SKD plan with the exception of higher counts of protein. You should be consuming additional carbs approximately 30 to 60 minutes before your workout times and follow the SKD plan at all other times. You will need to maintain the high-intensity exercise performance and promote the replacement of your glycogen at the same time without interrupting ketosis for long periods of time.

. . .

Two different types of people can benefit from the HPKD program. The first group of individuals who are just starting an exercise program and aren't ready to perform an abundance of exercises jobs to optimize the CKD diet plan. The second set of individuals that can use the plan are the ones using carbs to fuel their exercise performance, but cannot *or* will not take and carb loads of CKD. Just keep in mind that this CKD and the TKD plan are for individuals who are pushing their body to the limits and not just for craving suppression.

Two elements that occur when your body doesn't need the glucose:

Enter the Stage of Lipogenesis: If there is a sufficient supply of glycogen in your liver and muscles, any excess is converted to fat and stored.

Enter the Stage of Glycogenesis: The excess of glucose converts to glycogen and is stored in the muscles and liver. Research indicates that only about half of your energy used daily can be saved as glycogen. When the fatty acid molecules and glycerol are released, the ketogenesis process begins and creates acetoacetate.

The acetoacetate is changed into two types of ketone components:

- *Beta-hydroxybutyrate or BHB*: Your muscles will convert the acetoacetate into BHB which will fuel your brain after you have been on the keto diet for a short time.

- *Acetone:* This is mostly excreted as waste but can also be metabolized into glucose. This is the reason individuals on a ketogenic diet will experience a distinctive smelly breath.

When you enter ketosis, your body will have no more food. Thus, your body burns the fat to create ketones. Once the ketones break down the fats, which generate fatty acids, they will burn-off in the liver through beta-oxidation. Therefore, when you no longer have a supply of glycogen or glucose, ketosis begins and will use the stored fat as energy.

Use the keto calculator via the Internet at "keto-calculator.ankerl.-com." You can check your levels when you want to know what essentials your body needs during the course of your dieting plan or afterward. Just document your personal information such as height and weight into the calculator, and it will provide you with the essential math.

Know the Signs of Ketosis

. . .

You may experience several issues as you begin your new dieting strategies. These are a few just in case you have the problems, so you will know how to proceed.

Induction Flu is Present: The diet can make you irritable, nauseous, a bit confused, lethargic, and you may also suffer from a lingering headache. Several days into the plan should remedy these effects. If not, add one-half of a teaspoon of salt to a glass of water, and drink it to help with the side effects. However, you may need to do this once a day for about the first week, and it could take about 15-20 minutes before it helps. Relax, it will go away soon!

Leg Cramps: The loss of magnesium (a mineral) can be a factor that creates pain with the onset of the keto diet plan changes. With the loss of the minerals during urination, you could experience attacks of cramps in your legs.

Digestive Issues: You have made an enormous change in your diet overnight. It's expected that you may have problems including constipation or diarrhea when you first start the keto diet. This is yet another reason why you must drink plenty of water because you could quickly become constipated because of dehydration. The low-carbs contribute to the issue. Each person is different, and it will depend on what foods you have chosen to eat to increase your fiber intake. Try reducing new foods until the transitional phase of ketosis is concluded. It should clear up with time.

You may also be lacking beneficial bacteria. Try consuming fermented foods to increase your probiotics and aid digestion. You can benefit from B vitamins, omega 3 fatty acids, and beneficial enzymes as well. Eat the right veggies and add a small amount of salt to your food to help with the movements. Try a dose of *Milk of Magnesia.*

Heart Palpitations: You may begin to feel fluttery as a result of dehydration or because of an insufficient intake of salt. Try to adjust your menu plan by trying more carbs, but if you don't feel better quickly, you should seek emergency care.

Pungent Urine Smells: With the high acetone levels, your urine is also a strong indication to ketosis shown by its darkened color. There's no reason for concern; it's just your body adjusting to the new status.

Thirst is Increased: Fluid retention is increased when you are consuming carbohydrates. Once the carbs are flushed away, water weight is lost. If you are dehydrated; your body can use the stored carbs to restore hydration. When you're in ketosis, the carbs are removed, and your body doesn't have the water reserves. You need to realize that the keto state is a diuretic state, so drink plenty of water daily.

Keto Diet Benefits

The high-fat, low-carb diet plan offered by the ketogenic technique has been used by physicians since the 1920s to treat epilepsy. But with the onset of modern medicines, the ketogenic was vastly abandoned. However, in the past decade, it has begun to grow again as an effective therapy program for epileptic disorders.

. . .

S*eizure Reduction for Epilepsy Patients:* Reductions in seizures have occurred in children who use the ketogenic diet. The therapeutic keto diet used for epilepsy often restricts the carbs to fewer than 15 grams of carbs daily to further drive up the ketone levels. Don't try this unless you have the supervision of a medical professional.

D*ravet Syndrome:* Dravet Syndrome is a severe form of epilepsy which is marked by prolonged, uncontrollable, and frequent seizures which began in infancy. Medications that are available don't improve symptoms and approximately one-third of the Dravet Syndrome patients.

A clinical study used 13 children with Dravet Syndrome to stay on the ketogenic diet for more than one year to remain seizure-free. Over 50% of the group decreased in the frequency of the seizures. It was reported that six of the patients stopped the diet later, and one remains seizure-free.

I*mproved Thinking Skills:* Your brain is approximately 60% fat by weight. Therefore, you might become confused as you consume high-fat foods. By increasing your fatty foods intake; you will have better chances to better your mind. It can maintain itself and work at full capacity.

. . .

M*etabolic Syndrome Improved:* This is a collection of syndromes grouped together which enhances the risk of heart disease and diabetes. These include high blood sugar, high blood pressure, low HDL cholesterol, abdominal obesity, and high levels of triglycerides.

I*mprovement of your Cholesterol Profile:* An arterial buildup is generally associated with the triglyceride and cholesterol levels, which have been proven to improve with the keto diet plan.

L*ower Blood Pressures:* When you begin the ketogenic diet, your blood pressure may become lower making you feel dizzy at first. Don't worry or feel overly concerned because that's a clear indication that the carbohydrates are working. However, if you are currently taking medications, it's a good idea to speak with your physician about the possibility of lowering some of your doses while on the ketogenic diet plan.

I*mprovement & Reversal of Type 2 Diabetes:* Your blood sugar is brought to natural homeostasis as a result of the lowered amount of carbs that you're consuming. It's essential to understand that the carbohydrates stimulate the body's system to discharge the hormone called insulin. If you are not familiar with those with diabetes, it's the high amounts of blood sugar that comes primarily from your carbohydrate intake.

. . .

Once you have entered into a ketogenic diet, you will be eating fewer carbs. Therefore, your body can easily control the amount of blood sugar. Thus, when you lower your carb intake, your body doesn't release more insulin to control the blood sugar which in turn increase the burning of fat that has been stored in your body.

Improvements for Cancer: Initial research was provided by a cell biologist, Otto Warburg, who discovered that cancer cells flourish due to their ability to ferment glucose. Sugar is the primary source of food. Therefore, if you eliminate sugar from the diet, the cancer cells will become weakened and starve. More research is required, but the outlook is promising!

Polycystic Ovary Syndrome (PCOS) Improvement: This is an endocrine disorder affecting young women of childbearing years and is also associated with insulin resistance, obesity, and hyperinsulinemia. A 6-month study concluded a significant improvement in weight loss in fasting women over a 24-week period. The group limited carb intake to 20 grams daily for the 24 weeks.

Keto Diet Risks

A Word About Grapefruit: For 3.5 oz of pink, white, or red grapefruit is about 8 grams of net carbs. However, its benefits override the net carbs. The list is quite extensive since it promotes weight loss and fat burning, improves insulin resistance, it's low on the glycemic index, and low in calories. However, grapefruit may interact with some medications. It may not be the best combination since it has a lot of caffeine. It can slow down the elimination of caffeine from your body which can lead to overdose. Be sure to consult your physician first before using.

Iron Deficiencies: Iron is essential for the production of your red blood cells. The cells carry oxygen throughout the body. Once the levels become too low, there can be a deficiency in those cells with a condition called anemia. Anemia can cause pale skin, fatigue, and very thin or dull hair. It is recommended to consume iron-fortified cereal, oysters, beef, lentils, spinach, and beans; especially chickpeas, kidney beans, and white beans. Iron is essential for oxygen-rich blood.

Magnesium: It's fairly uncommon to experience a magnesium deficiency. It can affect those who have certain health conditions, who take certain medications or those who consume too much alcohol. It can also cause nausea, loss of appetite, fatigue, vomiting, weakness and more. In severe cases, it could lead to muscle cramps, numbness, abnormal heart rhythms, seizures, personality changes, or low potassium and calcium levels. Enjoy foods including cashews, almonds, spinach, peanuts, and black beans. Magnesium will help support your bone health and assist in energy production. The next time you're tired, have a dose of potassium.

Folate or Folic Acid: A deficiency in folate can cause symptoms including poor growth, mouth sores, fatigue, and change the color of the hair, skin, and nails. You can enjoy fortified cereals, leafy greens, lentils, and beans. The folic acid is extremely important for women of childbearing years. That's why it is a hefty dose in each prenatal vitamin.

You should speak to your doctor if you believe you have a nutrient deficiency. A blood test can determine the deficiency quickly. If the result is positive, and you do have a problem, a registered dietitian can recommend supplements for you. You could also take a multivitamin. Your physician will know what is best for your needs.

Calcium Deficiencies: Calcium is essential for maintaining your nerve function and muscle control as well as strong bones. It also strengthens your musculoskeletal system. Severely low calcium displays as abnormal heart rhythms and muscle cramps. Be sure you're getting plenty with at least three servings of yogurt or milk daily. You can also include calcium-fortified orange juice, dark leafy greens, and cheese. Just be sure they are keto friendly.

Vitamin D Deficiencies: Vitamin D is essential for maintaining strong bones. You can recognize a deficiency in vitamin D if you have symptoms of depression, increased blood pressure, muscle weakness, and bone pain. If you have limited sunshine in the winter time, this could also add to the deficiency. You can get vitamin D from three servings of yogurt or fortified milk daily. You can also eat tuna or salmon twice a week.

Adrenal Fatigue or Thyroid Disorder: It's possible to maintain a moderately low-carb diet such as keto if you have a thyroid condition such as hypothyroidism. You just need to keep a close check on the symptoms and reactions, especially if you are on other medications. If you notice the diet plan is worsening the symptoms, it's best to ask your physician. You could also consider increasing your carb intake by about 15 to 20 grams at a time until you find the desired amount you can use safely.

Potassium Deficiencies: It's possible for you to become low in potassium in the short-term because of the vomiting and diarrhea that could go along with your early stages to the keto plan. Symptoms of the deficiency could include constipation, muscle weakness, tingling and numbness, and a very severe case of abnormal heart rhythm.

However, there are other chronic conditions including kidney disease and eating disorders that could cause the deficiency. That's why it is so important to remain in contact with a physician during the dieting procedure. Natural potassium can also be received through milk, whole grains, bananas, veggies, peas, and beans.

As I stated earlier, these may not be a problem for you because everyone is different which means you may not have any issues with the new plan. But you know, an ounce of prevention is worth a pound of cure!

ULTIMATE DIET FOOD LIST

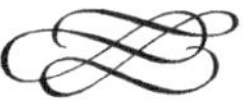

PLANNING AHEAD OF TIME ON YOUR KETOGENIC DIET MEANS you will be counting the carbs in the food you're planning to prepare. If you're starting from scratch and not using a recipe, you will want to know how many carbs you are consuming for each portion. You also need to understand some foods are not allowed on the diet plan.

Avoid These Foods

Some of these products may be used in your recipes in small amounts, but you should avoid these groups when you prepare your weekly meal plan.

Dairy Products: The ketogenic diet plan uses dairy and dairy products as an essential part of its planning. If you are lactose intolerant; maybe the keto plan isn't for you. It is suggested that you should not drink or consume more than four ounces daily. Choose dairy products that have been cultured and are keto-friendly. Serve and enjoy unsweetened almond milk, hemp milk, or flax milk. Avoid regular dairy since it packs almost 13 grams of carbohydrates per cup.

Artificial Sweeteners: Avoid several types including saccharin, sucralose, and Splenda.

Sugars to Avoid: Maltose, dextrose, honey, corn syrup, and maltodextrin should be avoided on the keto plan. These are how you could spend needless carbs:

- Honey: 17 g carbs
- Agave nectar: 16 g carbs
- White sugar: 12.6 g carbs
- Maple syrup: 13 g carbs

Avoid Juices: You will get a burst of energy from the juice but just a 12 oz. portion of unsweetened apple juice - packs 48 grams of carbohydrates. The delicious unsweetened grape juice passes that one for a 12 oz. serving - weighing in at 60 grams per serving – only 2 carbs from the fiber content. Keep in mind, that drinking juice can lead to hunger pangs and more unplanned snacking. It's probably easier to avoid it when possible.

Processed Foods: If you see carrageenan on the label, it's best to leave it on the shelf. Don't feel too guilty if you crave all of those processed foods. It happens!

Generally, look for labels with the least amount of ingredients. Usually, the ones that provide the most nutrition are listed in those shorter lists.

These are just a few examples of processed snacks to avoid while on a ketogenic diet. Some are surprising because they were deemed for years as a healthy and nutritious snack. I bet you see a few of the culprits that will beckon you onto the wrong path:

- Cereal Bars
- Rice cakes
- Flavored Nuts
- Popcorn
- Potato Chips
- Pretzels
- Protein Bars
- Crackers

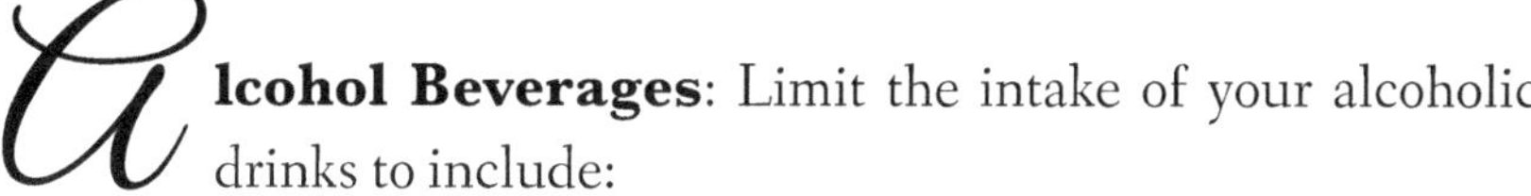

Alcohol Beverages: Limit the intake of your alcoholic drinks to include:

1. Cocktails
2. Flavored liquor
3. Beer
4. Dry Wine
5. Mixers: Soda, Juice, or Syrup

The keto professionals have deemed these spirits are acceptable:

- Vodka: Check the carb content since it is usually produced (grain-based) from potatoes, rye, and wheat

- Rum: Choose the ones with zero carbs or sugar.

- Whiskey, corn, barley, rye, and wheat are the grains used which have zero carbs or sugar.

- Tequila: The agave plant is the source of tequila.

S*pecial Note*: The alcohol listing doesn't promote you drinking alcohol, but alcohol does produce ketones in the liver. Remember, it still needs to be consumed in small amounts to prevent any detrimental health issues.

Healthy Food Choices

Purchase Fermented Foods

The natural acids found in fermented foods can help stabilize your blood sugar levels as well as the enzymes, probiotics, and other bioactive nutrients help support ketosis. These are excellent reasons you should consume fermented foods. Fermented foods help restore the 'good' bacteria in your gut.

- *Apple Cider Vinegar or ACV*: Many of your ketogenic recipes use vinegar. ACV also contains enzymes that can strengthen your immune system and enhance the metabolism of fats and proteins. It helps you lose weight and is a great energy booster. Use it for detoxification, reducing your cholesterol, helping to relieve sore muscles, and helping to balance your inner body system.

- *Yogurt:* Coconut milk is easily digested and contains fats including lauric acid. Yogurt provides transient bacteria since it feeds existing healthy gut bacteria as they pass through your intestinal tract.

- *Beet Kvass*: This slightly fizzy, earthy, slightly salty drink is a powerful healing tonic.

- *Natto* is a Japanese food product made from fermented soybeans. They are boiled and mixed with Bacillus subtilis (a bacteria culture). One cup will provide you with 50% of your daily recommended amounts of vitamin K. It's also a good source of calcium.

- *Miso* is a Japanese condiment that can promote good

heart health. Animal studies have indicated miso helps to reduce cholesterol in your blood.

- *Whole Eggs*. Visit your local area market for free-range options. You can scramble, fry, boil, or devil eggs up for a picnic or any occasion for a quick snack.

- *Grass-Fed Butter:* You can promote fat loss and butter is almost carb-free. The butter is a naturally occurring fatty acid which is rich in conjugated linoleic acid (CLA). It is suitable for maintaining weight loss and retaining lean muscle mass.

- *Ghee* is also a great staple for your keto stock which is also called clarified butter.

- *Kefir:* Health benefits include supporting detoxification, building your bone density, fighting off some types of cancer, and many other issues.

- *Heavy Whipping Cream*: This is an option almost unbelievable with only 5 grams of fat per tablespoon.

Include These Cold Items:

- Full-fat sour cream
- Goat cheese
- Full-fat cream cheese
- Parmesan cheese
- Hard & Soft cheeses – ex. mozzarella or sharp cheddar

Purchase Healthy Fats

Add Macadamia Oil: One of the benefits of this oil is that it has a high smoke point. It carries a mild flavor which is a super alternative to olive oil in mayonnaise.

Add Extra-Virgin Olive Oil (EVOO): Olive oil dates back for centuries to a time where oil was used for anointing kings and priests. High-quality oil with its low-acidity makes this oil have a smoke point as high as 410° Fahrenheit. That's higher than most cooking applications call for, making olive oil more heat-stable than many other cooking fats. It contains zero carbs for two teaspoons.

Monounsaturated fats, such as the ones in olive oil, are also linked with better blood sugar regulation, including lower fasting glucose, as well as reducing inflammation throughout the body. Olive oil also helps to prevent cardiovascular disease by protecting the integrity of your vascular system and lowering LDL which is also called the 'bad' cholesterol.

A*dd Coconut Oil:* You boost the fat intake with this high flash-point oil. Enjoy a coconut oil smoothie before your workouts. Use it with your meats, chicken, fish or on top of veggies. It will quickly transfer from solid form to oil according to its temperature.

Other Healthy Monounsaturated and Saturated Fats

Include these items (listed in grams):

- Olives – 3 jumbo - 5 large or 10 small – 1 gram of net carbs
- Avocado oil – 1 tbsp. -0- net carbs
- Chicken fat – 1 tbsp. -0- net carbs
- Duck Fat – 1 tbsp. -0- net carbs
- Beef Tallow – 1 tbsp. -0- net carbs
- Unsweetened flaked coconut – 3 tbsp. – 2 net carbs
- Unsalted Butter – 1 tbsp. -0- net carbs
- Ghee - 1 tsp. -0- net carbs
- Egg yolks – 1 large – 0.6 net carbs
- Organic Red Palm oil – ex. Nutivia - 1 tbsp. -0- net carbs
- Sesame oil – 1 tbsp. -0- net carbs
- Flaxseed oil – 1 tbsp. – 0 net carbs
- Various Dressings
- Keto-Friendly Mayonnaise

Load Up on Protein

Pastured Pork & Poultry: Choose from duck, pheasant, quail, or turkey breasts & ground turkey. Prepare chicken thighs, breasts, drumsticks, and ground chicken.

F*ish:* It is suggested by the dietary guidelines for Americans to consume at least 8 ounces of fish per week. It contains an abundance of vitamin D as well as healthy fat and protein. Fish and seafood are also good for your brain and will help with cognition and clarity while limiting the number of calories you're consuming.

It's preferable to eat fish that are caught in the wild. Include one single can of sardines (4 oz.) to receive 1,363 mg of omega-3 fatty acids and nearly 400 IU of vitamin D. You can also include fresh or canned tuna, trout, salmon, eel, catfish, flounder, cod, halibut, mahi-mahi, snapper, or mackerel as part of your diet plan. Just portion into bags and freeze until needed.

S*hellfish:* Choose crabs, clams, lobster, oysters, scallops, squid, shrimp, or mussels. Squid is 9 grams for .25 lb. Raw shrimp is 5 grams of net carbs for .25 lb. Imitation crab is 4.6 grams of net carbs for 1 ounce.

. . .

M*eat:* Grass-fed meats are preferred because they have a lower fatty acid count. Choose from veal, lamb, goat, or other wild game. Cuts of beef include chuck roast, flank steak, sirloin, or lean ground beef.

V*enison:* This is an excellent choice since it is lean, and is grass-raised meat.

N*uts & Seeds:* You can choose from an array of nuts in moderation. The

number of carbs represents the net carbs which equal approximately 3.5

ounces:

- Chia Seeds -0- grams
- Flax seeds -0- grams
- Brazil nuts – 4 grams
- Pecans – 4 grams
- Macadamia – 5 grams
- Hazelnuts – 7 grams
- Peanuts – 7 grams
- Walnuts – 7 grams
- Peanuts – 7 grams
- Pine Nuts – 9 grams
- Almonds – 10 grams
- Pumpkin seeds – 14.3 grams
- Sesame seeds – 17.7 grams
- Pistachios – 18 grams

M*ore About Fresh Seeds:* Pumpkin seeds are a great source of magnesium for you. They help immensely with your blood sugar levels and muscles. Flax seeds are another great source for omega-3 fatty acids. The micronutrients found in flax help reduce inflammation in your body. Psyllium seeds are also a good option. Coconut is also a good choice which can be used as shredded and unsweetened which weighs in at .25 cup for just 1.3 net carbs.

M*ore About Fresh Nuts:* Nuts have more minerals than many other foods. Brazil nuts are very high in selenium which is important for your immune system. It also assists your thyroid function. Walnuts are another great source of omega-3 fatty acids, protein, and fiber. The combo will fill you up and prevent blood sugar spikes. Almonds, hazelnuts, macadamia, pecans, pine nuts, cashews, or pistachios are also good choices.

Purchase Fresh Veggies

This list of veggies is excellent choices for your lunch or dinner menu plans. Each of these has the Net Carbs listed per 100 grams or 1/2 cup servings:

- Alfalfa Seeds – Sprouted - 0.2
- Arugula – 2.05
- Asparagus - 6 spears - 2.4
- Hass Avocado - ½ of 1 - 1.8

- Bamboo shoots - 3
- Beans – Green snap - 3.6
- Beet greens – 0.63
- Bell pepper -2.1
- Broccoli – 4.04
- Cabbage – Savoy – 3
- Carrots – 6.78
- Carrots – baby – 5.34
- Cauliflower – 2.97
- Celery – 1.37
- Chard – 2.14
- Chicory greens – 0.7
- Chives – 1.85
- Coriander – Cilantro leaves – 0.87
- Cucumber with peel – 3.13
- Eggplant – 2.88
- Garlic – 30.96
- Ginger root – 15.77
- Kale – 5.15
- Leeks – bulb (+) lower leaf – 12.35
- Lemongrass – citronella - 25.3
- Lettuce – red leaf – 1.36
- Lettuce – ex. iceberg - 1.77
- Mushrooms brown – 3.7
- Mustard Greens – 1.47
- Onions – yellow – 7.64
- Onions – scallions or spring – 4.74
- Onions – sweet – 6.65
- Peppers – banana – 1.95
- Peppers – red hot chili – 7.31
- Peppers – jalapeno – 3.7
- Peppers – sweet – green – 2.94

- Peppers – sweet – red – 3.93
- Peppers – sweet – yellow – 5.42
- Portabella mushrooms – 2.57
- Pumpkin – 6
- Radishes – 1.8
- Seaweed – kelp – 8.27
- Seaweed – spirulina - 2.02
- Shiitake mushrooms – 4.29
- Spinach – 1.43
- Squash – crookneck - summer – 2.64
- Squash – winter – acorn – 8.92
- Tomatoes – 2.69
- Turnips – 4.63
- Turnip greens – 3.93
- Summer squash - 2.6
- Raw watercress - 3.57
- White mushrooms – 2.26
- Zucchini - 1.5

Purchase Fresh Fruits

It's essential to eat plenty of fruits while on the keto diet plan. Add these choices according to your daily limits of carbohydrates. This collection of keto fruits are 100 grams or per 1/2 cup servings:

- Apples – no skin - boiled – 13.6 total carbs
- Apricots - 7.5 total carbs
- Bananas - 23.4 total carbs
- Fresh Blackberries - 5.4 net carbs
- Fresh Blueberries - 8.2 net carbs
- Fresh Strawberries - 3 net carbs

- Cantaloupe - 6 total carbs
- Raw Cranberries - 4 net carbs
- Gooseberries - 8.8 net carbs
- Kiwi – 14.2 total carbs
- Fresh Boysenberries - 8.8 net carbs
- Oranges – 11.7 total carbs
- Peaches - 11.6 total carbs
- Pears – 19.2 total carbs
- Pineapple - 11 total carbs
- Plums – 16.3 total carbs
- Watermelon- 7.1 total carbs

Lemon and Lime: These are two citric acid filled supplements to consider to help reduce your blood sugar levels naturally. The trace minerals in lemon and lime are present to improve your insulin—signaling a boost in your liver function. You can use them in many ways including overcooked veggies or meats, in your green juices, or with your salad to improve your state of ketosis.

Consider Ketogenic Sweetener Choices

Stevia Drops offer flavors including English toffee, hazelnut, vanilla, and chocolate. You can make sweetened coffee or other delicious drinks quickly. However, everyone is different, and some think the drops are bitter to taste. As a guideline, use three drops to equal one teaspoon of sugar.

. . .

Swerve Granular Sweetener is also an excellent choice as a blend made from non-digestible carbs sourced from starchy root veggies and select fruits. It's an excellent option for those who do not like the taste of stevia. Swerve is on the market as a one-to-one substitute. However, start with ¾ of a teaspoon for every one of sugar. Increase the portion as needed.

Swerve also has its own confectioners/powdered sugar for your baking needs. On the downside, it is more expensive than other products such as the Pyure.

Xylitol is on the topside of the sugary list. It is excellent for sweetening your teriyaki or BBQ sauce, and it does taste like sugar! The natural occurring sugar alcohol has the glycemic index (GI) standing of 13. Some have reported a slightly minty aftertaste. Xylitol is also known to keep your mouth bacteria in check and improving your dental health. It is commonly found in chewing gum. In large amounts, it can cause diarrhea - which gum can be considered as a laxative if used in large quantities.

Special Xylitol Warning: If you have a puppy in the house that enjoys investigating and tasting everything, be sure to use caution since it is toxic to dogs - even small amounts.

Begin with Healthy Spices

Black Pepper (.0 grams) Pepper promotes nutrient absorption in the tissues all over your body, speeds up your metabolism, and improves digestion. The main ingredient of pepper is a pipeline which gives it the pungent taste. It can boost fat metabolism by as much as 8% for up to several hours after it's ingested. As you will see, it's used in many of your ketogenic recipes.

H*imalayan Pink Salt* (.0 grams) has an abundance of essential minerals required by the human body and promotes a healthy pH balance of the cells. It is also a good source of magnesium which has an overall 80% deficiency in all individuals.

B*asil* (0.1 grams per 2 tbsp.) You can use fresh or dried basil to maximize its benefits. Its dark green color is an indication it also maintains an outstanding source of magnesium, calcium, and vitamin K which is excellent for your bones. It also helps with allergies, arthritis or inflammatory bowel conditions.

C*ayenne Pepper* (3 grams per tbsp.) The secret ingredient in cayenne is the capsaicin which is a natural compound that gives the peppers their fiery heat. This provides a short increase in your metabolism. The peppers are also rich in vitamins, effective as an appetite controller, smooths out digestion issues, and benefits your heart health.

Turmeric: (6.3 carbs per 1 tbsp.) The use or this Asian orange herb dates back to Ayurveda and Chinese medicine. The curcumin which is an anti-inflammatory compound found in the turmeric helps improve your insulin receptor function while regulating your blood sugar levels. It aids in digestion and improves weight management. Add turmeric to your meats, vegetables, green drinks, or smoothies.

Ground Chia Seeds: (.77 grams per 3.5 oz.) The seeds are gluten-free and can absorb up to 11 times its weight in liquid. Be sure to add plenty of water and soak them for at least 5 minutes before using in your keto recipes. Otherwise, you will have some uncomfortable digestion after eating them. Be sure to remain hydrated.

Cinnamon (6 grams per 1 tbsp.) Use cinnamon as part of your daily plan to improve your insulin receptor activity. Just put one-half of a teaspoon of cinnamon into a smoothie, shake, or any other keto dessert. As you will observe, many of the keto recipes contain the ingredient.

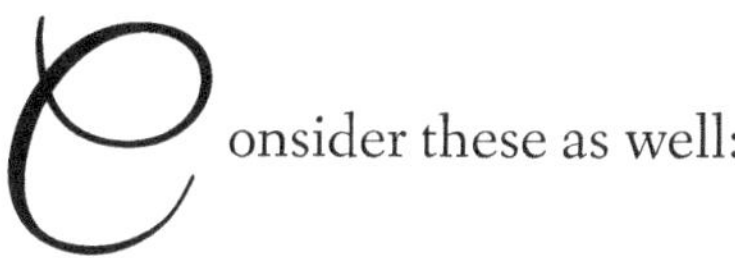

Consider these as well:

- *Garlic Powder* (7 grams per 1 tbsp.)
- *Nutmeg* (3.5 grams per 1 tbsp.)
- *Paprika* (3.7 grams per 1 tbsp.)
- *Thyme* (0.2 grams per tsp.)
- *Dill Seed* (3.6 grams per 1 tbsp.)

Make Your Homemade Pumpkin Pie Spice: Use this simple low-carb concoction, and you know it will be healthy.

Servings: 10.75 tsp. @ 1 tsp. per serving

Total Macros:

- 0.8 g Net Carbs
- 0.09 g Fat
- 0.12 g Protein
- 6.42 Calories

Ingredients:

- Ground cinnamon (2 tbsp.)
- Ground nutmeg (.5 tsp.)
- Ground ginger (1 tbsp.)
- Allspice (.5 tsp.)
- Cardamom (.25 tsp.)
- Ground cloves (.5 tsp. or .75 tsp. whole cloves)

Preparation Instructions:

1. Use a spice grinder to grind the cloves into powder.
2. Combine all of the components into a large mixing container until combined thoroughly.
3. Store in a spice container to use any time the need arises.

Make Your Homemade Poultry Seasoning:

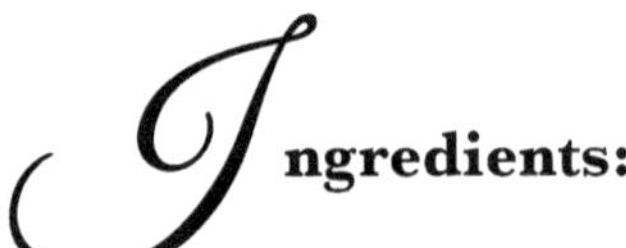

ngredients:

- Dried sage (2 tbsp.)
- Dried marjoram (1 tbsp.)
- Ground nutmeg (.5 tbsp.)
- Dried rosemary (.5 tbsp.)
- Dried thyme (1.5 tbsp.)
- Ground black pepper (.5 tbsp.)

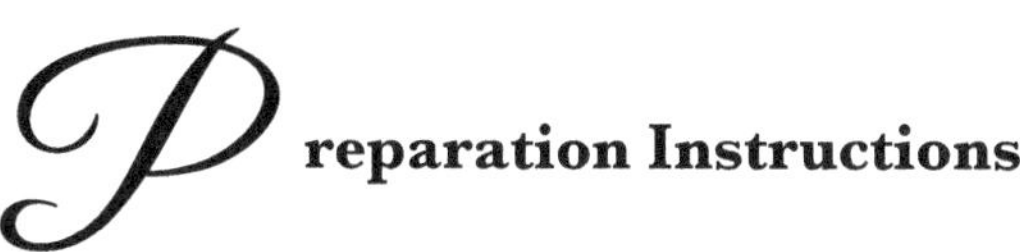

Preparation Instructions:

1. Mix each of the spices in a small jar or another type of storage container.
2. Use freely any time you want a little kick to your poultry.

A Word About Flour

Transitioning into the ketogenic way of living can be made easier by using low-carb substitutions for common goods used in cooking and baking. These are just a few ways keto-friendly products that can be used to save the carbohydrates and provide you with an alternative plan.

Coconut Flour: You can use coconut flour in many of the keto diet meals. When using coconut flour, remember it isn't a 1:1 ratio. In comparison, you can substitute as little as 1/3 cup to 1/4 cup of coconut flour. Use one-part water to one-part coconut flour and whisk together to use as a thickening agent. Just add it to hot liquids such as soup. It's high in fiber - making it super absorbent. You can add oils, eggs, and other liquids as needed. Use the coconut flour at times you are sautéing or frying foods.

Almond Flour: Almond flour is a suitable replacement and is used as all-purpose flour. Each one-quarter cup portion is only 3 carbohydrates per gram. The process involves blanching the almonds in boiling water to remove the skins. Next, you will grind the flour into a finely ground product that is an excellent choice for cakes, cookies, and pie crusts.

Sesame Flour: Finely grind sesame seeds to prepare the flour into a texture similar to wheat flour. Combine with psyllium flour for your baking needs to ensure the light texture of high-carb white bread.

Whole Psyllium Husk: Use the entire husk in doughs where you require more 'stretchiness' such as what you would have in wheat flour. It's excellent for pizza dough, tortillas, or bread.

Psyllium Husk Powder: Fiber is its main ingredient, but it is combined with other low-carb flours.

KETO BREAKFAST & BRUNCH RECIPES

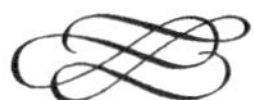

GET YOUR MORNING OFF TO A GREAT START WITH ONE OF these delicious meals.

Almost "McGriddle" Casserole

**ervings**: 8

Total Macros:

- 3 g Net Carbs
- 36 g Fat
- 26 g Protein
- 448 Calories

Ingredients:

- Breakfast sausage (1 lb.)
- Flaxseed meal (.25 cup)
- Almond flour (1 cup)
- Large eggs (10)
- Maple syrup (6 tbsp.)
- Cheese (4 oz.)
- Butter (4 tbsp.)
- Onion (.5 tsp.)
- Garlic powder (.5 tsp.)
- Sage (.25 tsp.)
- Also Needed: 9 x 9-inch casserole dish

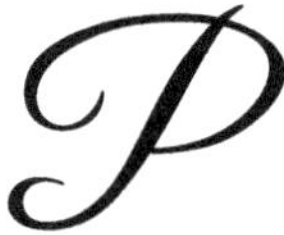

reparation Instructions:

1. Warm up the oven temperature to reach 350° Fahrenheit. Prepare the casserole dish with a sheet of parchment paper.
2. Use the medium heat setting on the stovetop to cook the sausage in a skillet.
3. Add all of the dry ingredients (the cheese also), and stir in the wet ones.
4. Add 4 tablespoons of the syrup. Stir and blend well.
5. After the sausage is browned, combine all of the fixings along with the grease.

6. Empty the mix into the casserole dish and drizzle the rest of the syrup on the top.
7. Bake for 45-55 minutes.
8. Transfer to the countertop until it's room temperature.
9. The casserole should be easy to remove by using the edge of the parchment paper. After the casserole has cooled; just slice it into 8 portions.

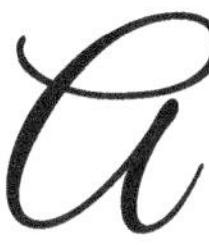

Avocado & Bacon Omelet

Servings: 1

Total Macros:

- 3.3 g Net Carbs
- 63 g Fat
- 30 g Protein
- 719 Calories

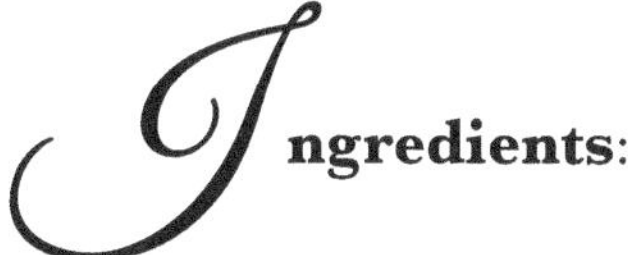

Ingredients:

- Crispy bacon (1 slice)
- Large organic eggs (2)
- Freshly grated parmesan cheese (.5 cup)
- Ghee or coconut oil or butter (2 tbsp.)
- Salt (1 pinch)
- Avocado (.5 of 1 small)

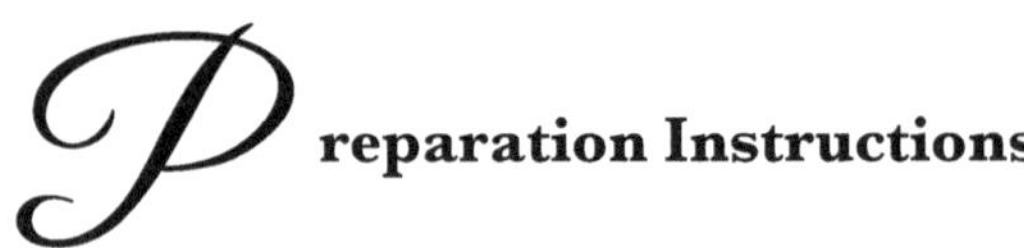

Preparation Instructions:

1. Cook the bacon and set aside.
2. Combine the eggs with the parmesan cheese and your choice of finely chopped herbs.
3. Heat up a skillet and add the butter/ghee to melt using the medium-high heat setting.
4. When hot, whisk and add the eggs. Prepare the omelet working it towards the middle of the pan for about 30 seconds. When firm, flip and cook for another 30 seconds.
5. Arrange on a plate and garnish with the crunched bacon bits. Serve with the sliced avocado**.**

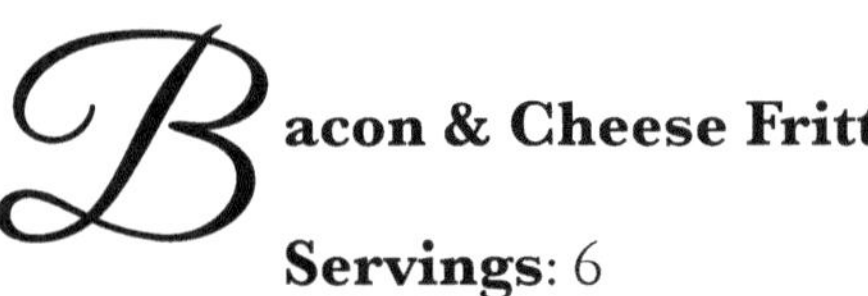

Bacon & Cheese Frittata

Servings: 6

Total Macros:

- 2 g Net Carbs
- 29 g Fat
- 13 g Protein
- 320 Calories

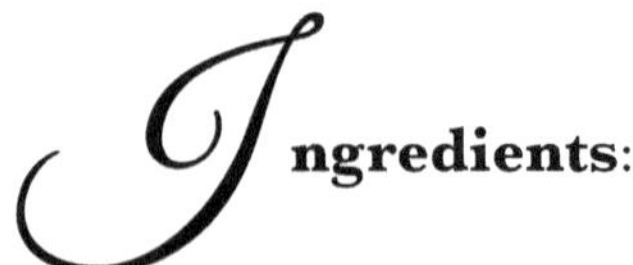

Ingredients:

- Heavy cream (1 cup)
- Eggs (6)
- Black pepper (.25 tsp.)
- Crispy slices of bacon (5)
- Chopped green onions (2)
- Cheddar cheese (4 oz.)
- Salt (.5 tsp.)
- Also Needed: 1 pie plate

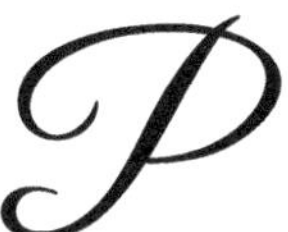**reparation Instructions**:

1. Heat up the oven temperature setting to 350° Fahrenheit.
2. Whisk the eggs and seasonings. Empty into the pie pan and top off with the rest of the fixings.
3. Bake 30-35 minutes. Let the cake rest for a few minutes before serving for the best results.

Blueberry Ricotta Pancakes

Servings: 5

Total Macros:

- 6 g Net Carbs
- 23 g Fat
- 15 g Protein
- 311 Calories

Ingredients Needed:

- Ricotta (.75 cup)
- Large eggs (3)
- Unsweetened vanilla almond milk (.25 cup)
- Golden flaxseed meal (.5 cup)
- Salt (.25 tsp.)
- Baking powder (1 tsp.)
- Almond flour (1 cup)
- Stevia powder (.5 tsp.)
- Vanilla extract (.5 tsp.)
- Blueberries (.25 cup)
- Optional: Keto-friendly syrup of choice

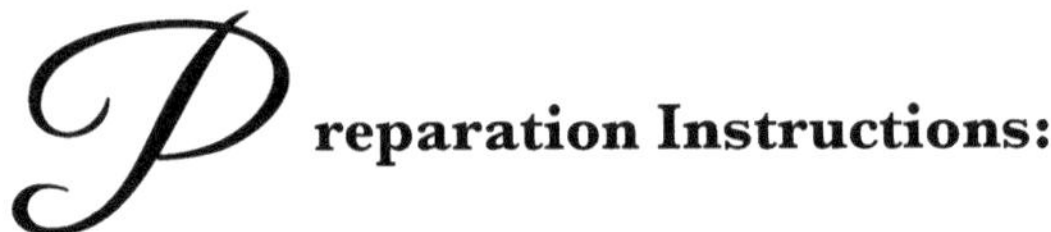

Preparation Instructions:

1. Blend the eggs, milk, ricotta, and vanilla extract with an electric mixer.
2. Combine the flaxseed meal, salt, flour, baking powder, and stevia in another dish.
3. Add the dry ingredients into the blender—slowly—to form the batter. Use two to three blueberries for each pancake.
4. Add the butter to a preheated skillet using the medium heat setting. When it melts, add the batter using two

tablespoons for each scoop.

5. At this point, serve or set aside to cool.
6. You can serve or freeze to use later if you have limited time. If you know your schedule will be rushed; you can pour the syrup in a cup with a lid.
7. Serve with a side of bacon but add the additional carbs.

elicious Fully Herbed 'Fatty' Omelet

Servings: 1

Total Macros:

- 3.3 g Net Carbs
- 63 g Fat
- 30 g Protein
- 719 Calories

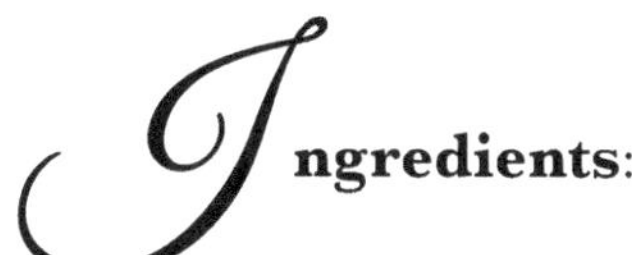

ngredients:

- Large eggs (2)
- Grated parmesan cheese (.5 cup)
- Freshly chopped basil (1 tbsp.)
- Ghee (2 tbsp.)
- Freshly chopped oregano (.5 tbsp.)
- Salt (1 pinch)
- Crispy bacon (1 slice)

- Small avocado (.5 of 1)

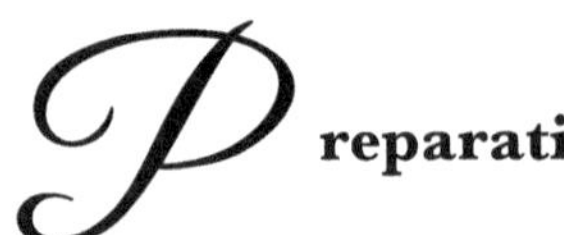**reparation Instructions**:

1. Grate the parmesan. Whisk the eggs with the parmesan and herbs. Stir in the oregano and basil.
2. Warm up a skillet with a spritz of oil using the med-high heat setting. Add the egg and reduce the heat setting to medium.
3. For the first 30 seconds, bring the egg to the center of the pan with a spatula. Once the top is firm; flip and cook about 30 seconds.
4. Serve with a topping of sliced avocado and crispy bacon.

Lavender Biscuits

Servings: 6

Total Macros:

- 4 g Net Carbs
- 25 g Fat
- 10 g Protein
- 270 Calories

Ingredients:

- Coconut oil (.33 cup)
- Almond flour (1.5 cups)
- Egg whites (4)
- Kosher salt (1 pinch)
- Baking powder (1 tsp.)
- Culinary grade lavender buds (1 tbsp.)
- Liquid stevia (4 drops)

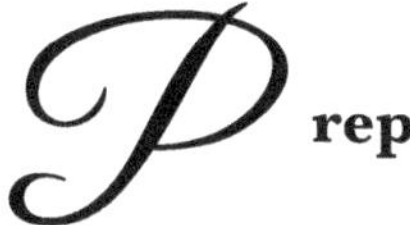

Preparation Instructions:

1. Warm up the oven until it reaches 350° Fahrenheit. Spritz a baking sheet with a little coconut oil.
2. Combine the almond flour and coconut oil in a mixing container until it's pea-sized pieces. Set the bowl aside in the fridge.
3. Whisk the eggs until they start foaming. Toss in the salt, lavender, and baking powder. Stir well and mix in the eggs. Mix in with the almond mixture, stirring well.
4. Place the biscuits onto the baking sheet using an ice cream scoop or tablespoon. Pat them, so they aren't round similar to a pancake.
5. Bake for 20 minutes and serve.

Mackerel & Egg Plate for Brunch

Servings: 2

Total Macros:

- 4 g Net Carbs
- 59 g Fat
- 35 g Protein
- 689 Calories

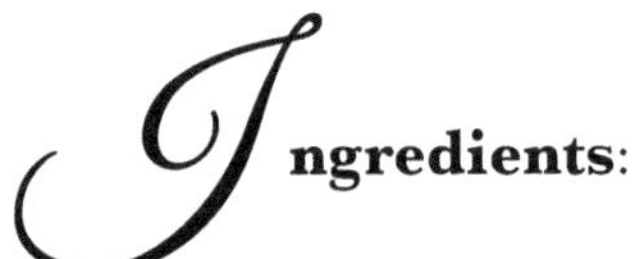

Ingredients:

- Eggs (4)
- Butter for frying (2 tbsp.)
- Canned mackerel in tomato sauce (8 oz.)
- Lettuce (2 oz.)
- Red onion (.5 of 1)
- Olive oil (.25 cup)
- Salt and pepper (to your liking)

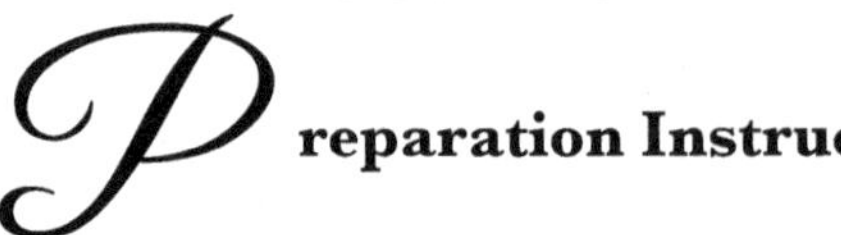

Preparation Instructions:

1. Warm up the frying pan and prepare your eggs in the butter.

2. Add lettuce to a platter and layer with the onion and mackerel. Place the eggs to the side and season with salt and pepper to your liking.
3. Spritz the oil over the salad and serve.

Mushroom Omelet

Servings: 1

Total Macros:

- 4 g Net Carbs
- 43 g Fat
- 25 g Protein
- 510 Calories

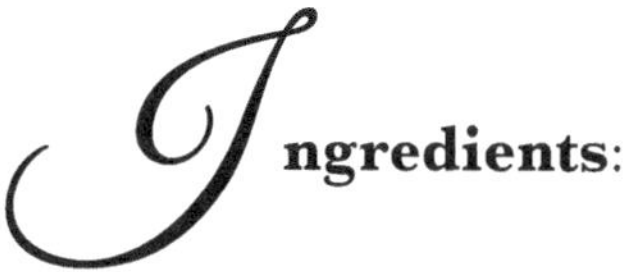

Ingredients:

- Butter (1 oz.)
- Eggs (3)
- Shredded cheese (1 oz.)
- Yellow onion (3 tbsp.)
- Mushrooms (3)
- Pepper and Salt (to taste)

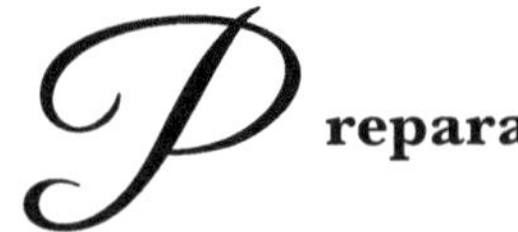

reparation Instructions:

1. Whisk the eggs with the salt and pepper until frothy.
2. Sprinkle in the spices.
3. Add the butter to a skillet. When melted, add the eggs.
4. Prepare the omelet. Once the bottom is firm, sprinkle with the onions, mushrooms, and cheese.
5. Carefully, remove the edges and fold the omelet in half.
6. Slide onto the plate when done.

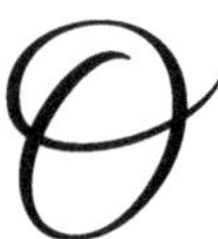

ven-Baked Pancake with Onions & Bacon

Servings: 4

Total Macros:

- 5 g Net Carbs
- 50 g Fat
- 16 g Protein
- 545 Calories

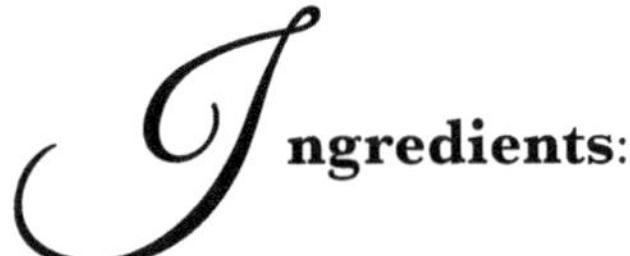

ngredients:

- Turkey or pork bacon (3.5 oz.)

- Yellow onion (.5 of 1)
- Butter to fry in (2 tbsp.)
- Eggs (4)
- Heavy whipping cream (1 cup)
- Cottage cheese (.5 cup)
- Almond flour (.5 cup)
- Ground psyllium husk powder (1 tbsp.)
- Baking powder (1 tsp.)
- Salt (1 tsp.)
- Optional: Chopped fresh parsley - for garnish (1 tbsp.)

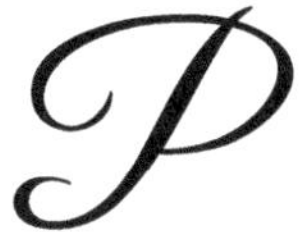

Preparation Instructions:

1. Warm up the oven to reach 350° Fahrenheit. Chop the onion and bacon.
2. Prepare a skillet and add the onion until they start crisping. Set aside.
3. Whisk the eggs, cream, and cottage cheese. Mix in with the baking powder, psyllium husk, salt, and almond flour. Let it rest for 2-3 minutes.
4. Add the batter to the prepared pan and sprinkle with the crispy onion and bacon.
5. Bake until the center is set or about 20-25 minutes.

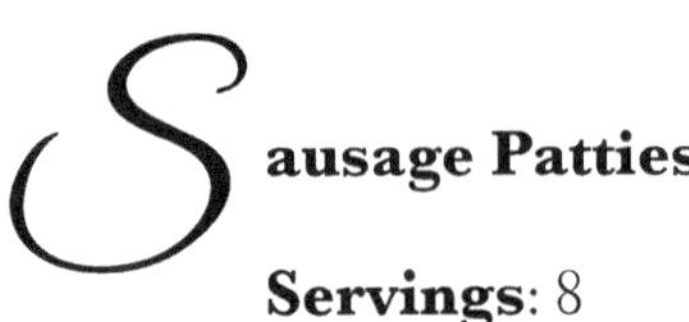

ausage Patties

Servings: 8

Total Macros:

- 1.4 g Net Carbs
- 11 g Fat
- 21 g Protein
- 187 Calories

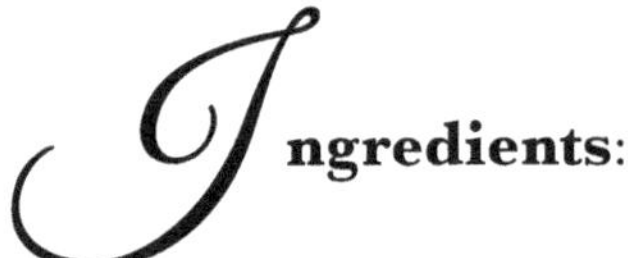

ngredients:

- Maple extract (1 tsp.)
- Granular swerve sweetener (2 tbsp.)
- Garlic powder (.25 tsp.)
- Pepper (.5 tsp)
- Cayenne (.125 tsp.)
- Salt (1 tsp.)
- Freshly chopped sage (2 tbsp.)
- Ground pork (1 lb.)
- For the Pan: Olive oil (1 tsp.)

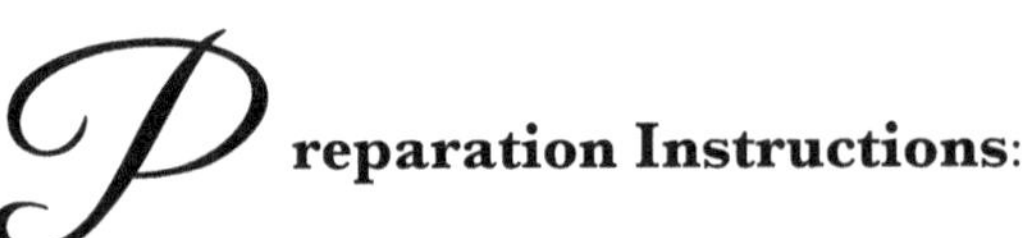

reparation Instructions:

1. Whisk each of the fixings in a mixing container and add the pork. Mix well.
2. Shape the patties to approximately a one-inch thickness.
3. Add the olive oil or some of the butter to a pan on the stovetop using the medium heat setting. Cook each side for three to four minutes.

KETO LUNCH FAVORITES

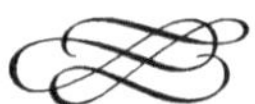

Salad Favorites

BLT In A Jar

Servings: 8

Total Macros:

- 7 g Net Carbs
- 18 g Fat
- 17 g Protein
- 205 Calories

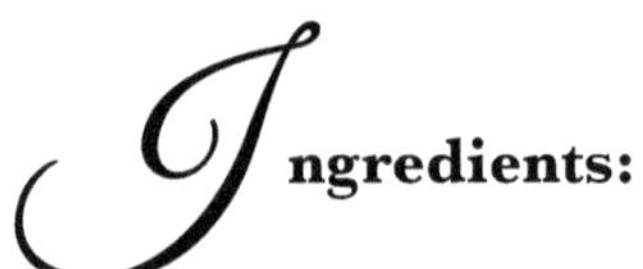

ngredients:

- Romaine Lettuce (2 cups)
- Iceberg Lettuce (2 cups)
- Chopped scallions (2)
- Diced tomatoes (2)
- Bacon slices (4 crumbled)

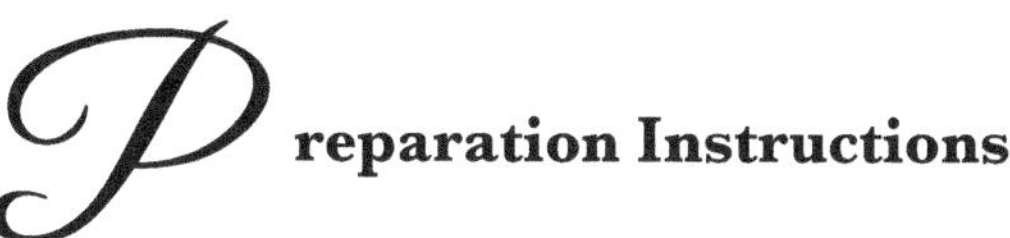

Preparation Instructions:

1. Combine all of the dressing components.
2. Slowly pour into the jars.
3. Layer the veggies, croutons, and add a garnish of bacon.
4. Tightly close each of the jars.
5. Store in the fridge for up to three days.

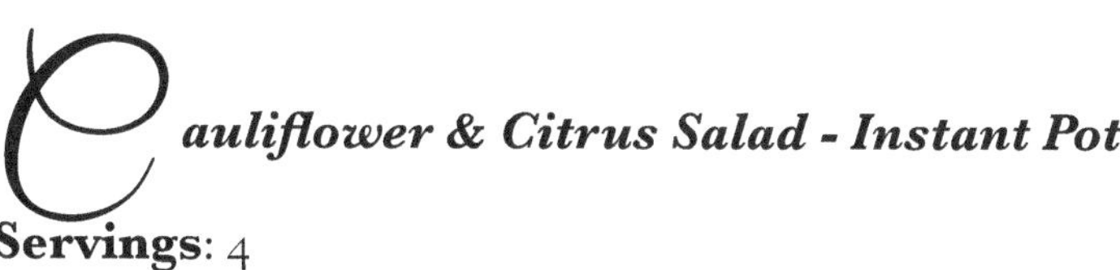

Cauliflower & Citrus Salad - Instant Pot

Servings: 4

Total Macros:

- 1 g Net Carbs
- 7 g Fat
- 2 g Protein
- 177 Calories

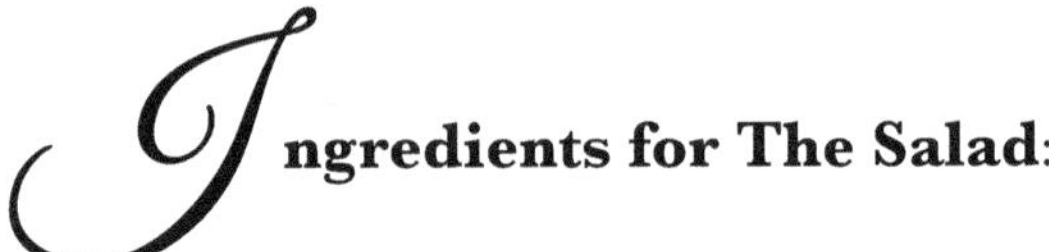

Ingredients for The Salad:

- Small cauliflower (1 - divided)
- Small Romanesco cauliflower (1 - divided)
- Broccoli (1 lb.)
- Seedless oranges (2)

Ingredients for The Vinaigrette:

- Finely chopped anchovies (4)
- Orange juice & zest (1)
- Salted – unrinsed capers (1 tbsp.)
- Finely chopped hot pepper (1)
- Pepper & Salt (to your liking)
- Extra-virgin olive oil (4 tbsp.)

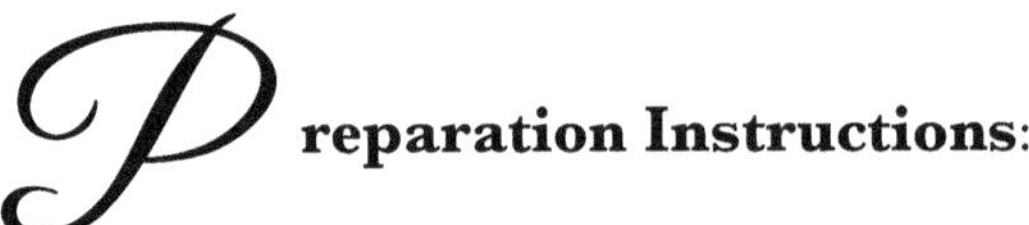

Preparation Instructions:

1. Cut the cauliflower into florets. Remove the peel and thinly slice the oranges. Finely chop the anchovies, capers, and hot peppers for the vinaigrette.

2. Prepare the vinaigrette fixings in a jar with a lid. Shake well and set aside.
3. Set up the Instant Pot with one cup of water and the steamer basket. Add the cauliflower to the basket and secure the lid. Set the timer for 6 minutes using low pressure. Quick-release the steam pressure when you hear the buzzer.
4. Transfer the florets to a serving dish with the prepared oranges. Toss.
5. Drizzle with the vinaigrette and serve.

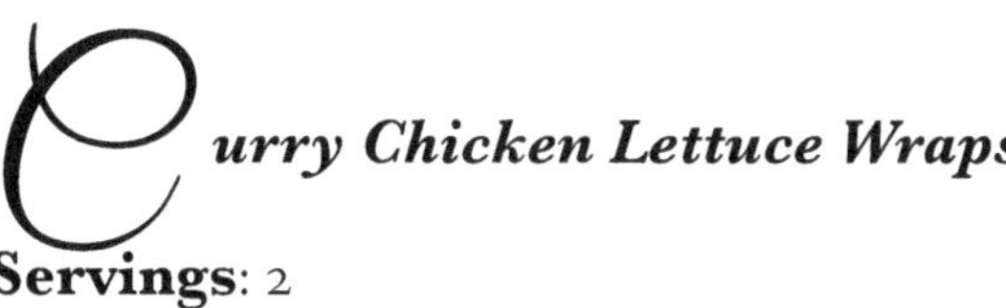

urry Chicken Lettuce Wraps

Servings: 2

Total Macros:

- 7 g Net Carbs
- 36 g Fat
- 50 g Protein
- 554 Calories

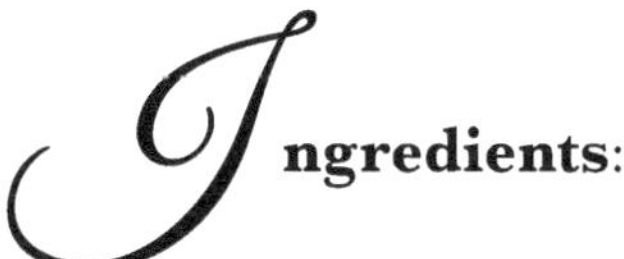

ngredients:

- Minced onion (.25 cup)
- Ghee (3 tbsp.)
- Chicken thighs – skinless & boneless (1 lb.)

- Black pepper (1 tsp.)
- Minced garlic cloves (2)
- Salt (1.5 tsp.)
- Curry powder (2 tsp.)
- Riced cauliflower (1 cup)
- Lettuce leaves (5-6)
- Keto-friendly sour cream (as desired - count the carbs)

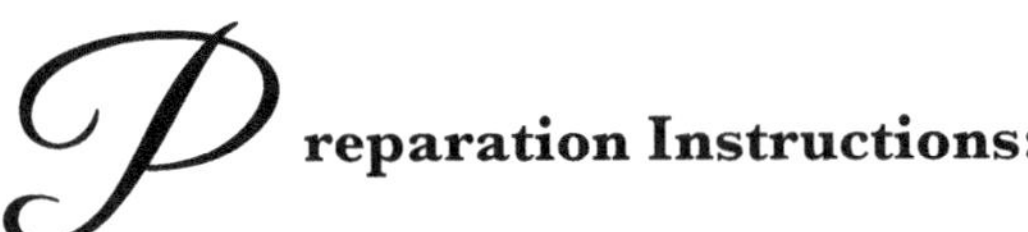

Preparation Instructions:

1. Mince the garlic and onions. Set aside for now.
2. Remove the skin and bones from the chicken and chop into 1-inch pieces.
3. On the stovetop, add 2 tbsp. of the ghee to a skillet and melt. Toss in the onion and sauté until browned. Fold in the chicken and sprinkle with the garlic, pepper, and salt.
4. Cook for eight minutes. Stir in the remainder of the ghee, riced cauliflower, and curry. Stir until well mixed.
5. Prepare the lettuce leaves and add the mixture.
6. Serve with a dollop of cream.

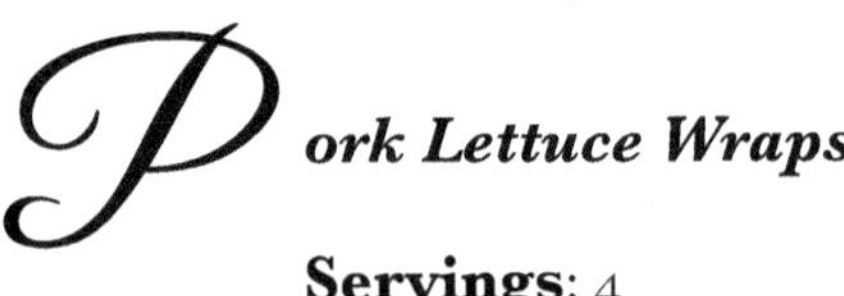

Pork Lettuce Wraps

Servings: 4

Total Macros:

- 7 g Net Carbs
- 24 g Fat

- 23 g Protein
- 340 Calories

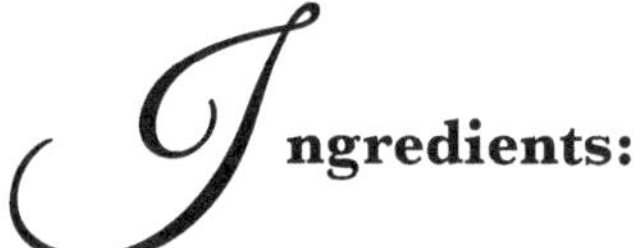

Ingredients:

- Sesame oil - divided (4 tbsp.)
- Olive oil (2 tbsp.)
- Thinly sliced pork (1 lb.)
- Minced garlic cloves (2)
- Chili garlic sauce (1 tsp.)
- Gluten-free soy sauce or another keto-friendly choice (2-3 tbsp.)
- Rice wine vinegar (2-3 tbsp.)
- Large julienned carrot (1)
- Large julienned cucumber (.5 of 1)
- Freshly chopped cilantro (2 tbsp.)
- Small head romaine lettuce (1)

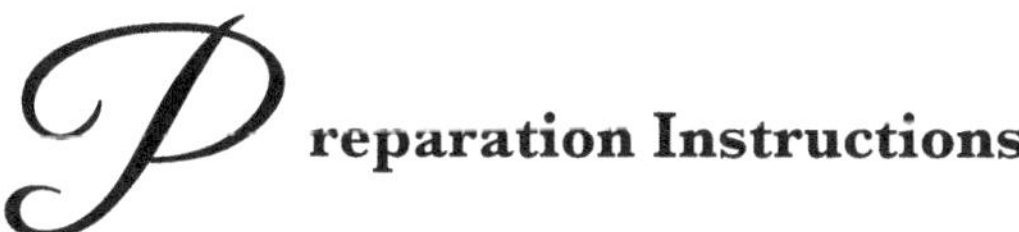

Preparation Instructions:

1. Warm the olive oil in a skillet using the medium temperature setting. Toss in the garlic and sauté for one to two minutes.
2. Stir in 2 tablespoons of the sesame oil and the pork.

Prepare until crispy (5-6 min.). Set it aside for now.

3. In a small container, mix the rest of the sesame oil, vinegar, chili garlic sauce, and soy sauce.
4. Stir in the cucumber and carrot with the dressing. Toss well.
5. Assemble the wraps. Prepare the lettuce cups with a layer of pork and vegetables.
6. Serve with a portion of fresh cilantro.

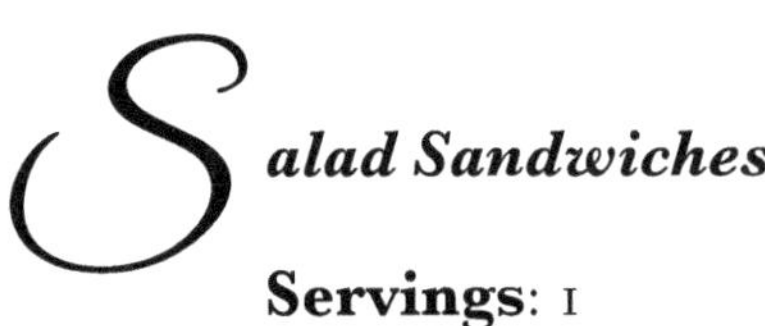

alad Sandwiches

Servings: 1

Total Macros:

- 3 g Net Carbs
- 34 g Fat
- 10 g Protein
- 374 Calories

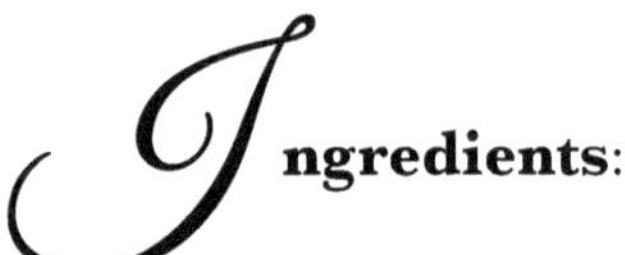

ngredients:

- Romaine lettuce (2 oz.)
- Butter (.5 oz.)
- Edam or your favorite cheese (1 oz.)
- Cherry tomato (1)
- Avocado (.5 of 1)

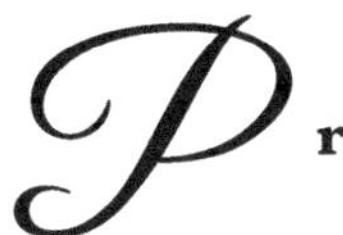

reparation Instructions:

1. Rinse the lettuce and drain in a colander.
2. Add the lettuce to a salad dish and smear with the butter, slice of cheese, avocado slices, and the tomato on top.
3. Serve any time for a delicious meal or snack.

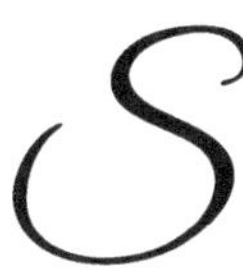

wedish Shrimp Salad with Dill

Servings: 4

Total Macros:

- 2 g Net Carbs
- 48 g Fat
- 14 g Protein
- 496 Calories

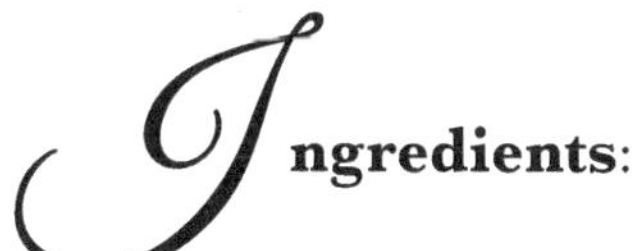

ngredients:

- Shrimp, peeled and cooked (10 oz.)
- Mayonnaise (1 cup)
- Sour cream or crème fraiche (.25 cup)

- Fresh dill (2 tbsp.)
- Fish roe (2 oz.)
- Lemon juice (2 tsp.)
- Salt and pepper (as desired)

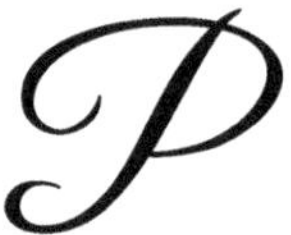

reparation Instructions:

1. Roughly chop half of the shrimp.
2. Combine the sour cream and mayonnaise in a mixing container.
3. Fold in the dill, roe, and shrimp. Reserve a portion for garnishing.
4. Sprinkle with the pepper and salt.
5. Drizzle with the lemon juice before serving.

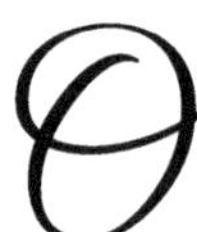

ther Choices

Cheeseburger Calzone

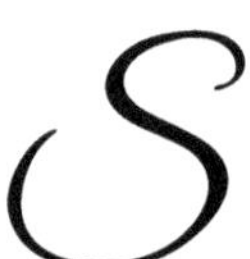

ervings: 8

Total Macros:

- 3 g Net Carbs
- 47 g Fat
- 34 g Protein

- 580 Calories

Ingredients:

- Dill pickle spears (4)
- Cream cheese – divided (8 oz.)
- Shredded mozzarella cheese (1 cup)
- Egg (1)
- Yellow diced onion (.5 of 1)
- Ground beef - lean (1.5 lb.)
- Thick-cut bacon strips (4)
- Mayonnaise (.5 cup)
- Shredded cheddar cheese (1 cup)
- Almond flour (1 cup)

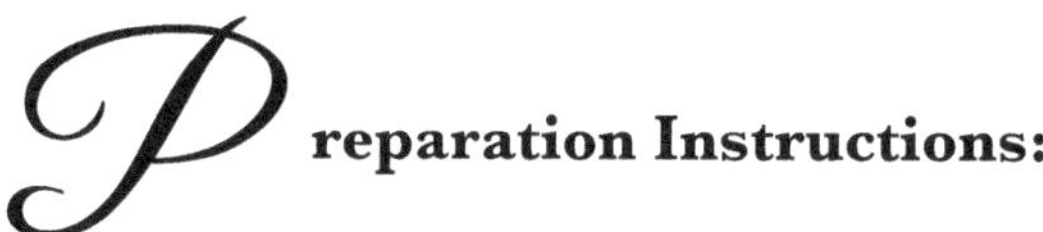

Preparation Instructions:

1. Program the oven temperature setting to 425° Fahrenheit. Prepare a cookie tin with parchment paper.
2. Chop the pickles into spears. Set aside for now.
3. Prepare the crust. Combine ½ of the cream cheese and the mozzarella cheese. Microwave for 35 seconds. When it melts, add the egg and almond flour to make the dough. Set aside.

4. Cook the beef on the stove using the medium heat setting.
5. Cook the bacon until crunchy (microwave for five minutes or stovetop). When cool, break into bits.
6. Dice the onion and add to the beef. Cook until softened. Toss in the bacon, cheddar cheese, pickle bits, the rest of the cream cheese, and mayonnaise. Stir well.
7. Roll the dough onto the prepared baking tin. Scoop the mixture into the center. Fold the ends and side to make the calzone.
8. Bake until browned for about 15 minutes. Let it rest for 10 minutes before slicing.

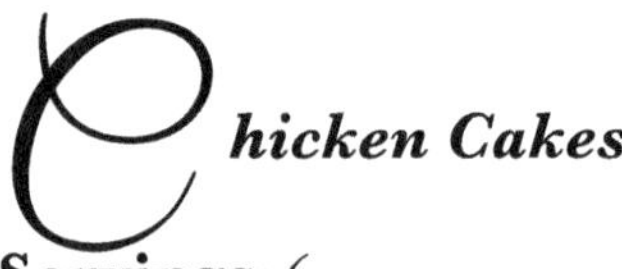

hicken Cakes

Servings: 6

Total Macros:

- 3.7 g Net Carbs
- 15.6 g Fat
- 12.8 g Protein
- 203 Calories

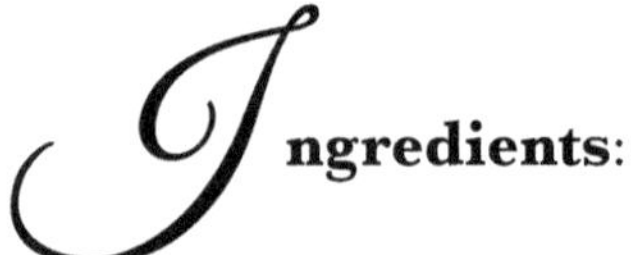

ngredients:

- Eggs (3)

- Ground chicken (6 oz.)
- Rosemary (1 tsp.)
- Salt (.5 tsp.)
- Basil (1 tsp.)
- Coconut flour (3 tbsp.)
- Almond flour (.25 cup)
- Butter (2 tbsp.)
- Almond milk (.5 cup)

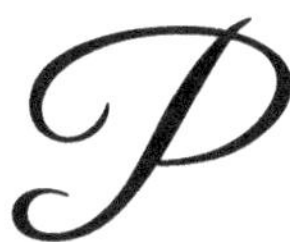

reparation Instructions:

1. Whisk the eggs and stir in the rosemary, salt, and basil. Stir in the almond milk using a hand mixer.
2. Mix in both of the flours to make a soft dough. Fold in the ground chicken using a wooden spoon.
3. Warm up a skillet with the butter. Prepare six servings. Cook two minutes per side. Serve hot.

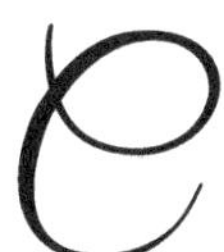

hicken "Zoodle" Soup

Servings: 2

Total Macros:

- 4 g Net Carbs
- 16 g Fat
- 34 g Protein

- 310 Calories

Ingredients:

- Chicken broth (3 cups)
- Chicken breast (1)
- Avocado oil (2 tbsp.)
- Green onion (1)
- Celery stalk (1)
- Cilantro (.25 cup)
- Salt (to your liking)
- Zucchini (1)

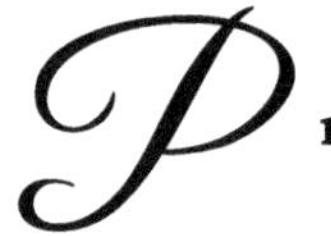

reparation Instructions:

1. Chop or dice the breast of the chicken. Pour the oil into a saucepan and cook the chicken until done. Pour in the broth and simmer. Chop the celery and green onions and toss into the pan. Simmer for 3-4 more minutes.
2. Chop the cilantro and prepare the zucchini noodles. Use a spiralizer or potato peeler to make the 'noodles.' (Remove the peel.) Add to the pot.
3. Simmer for a few more minutes and season to your liking.
4. Store in a glass container in the fridge. It will remain tasty for 2-3 days.

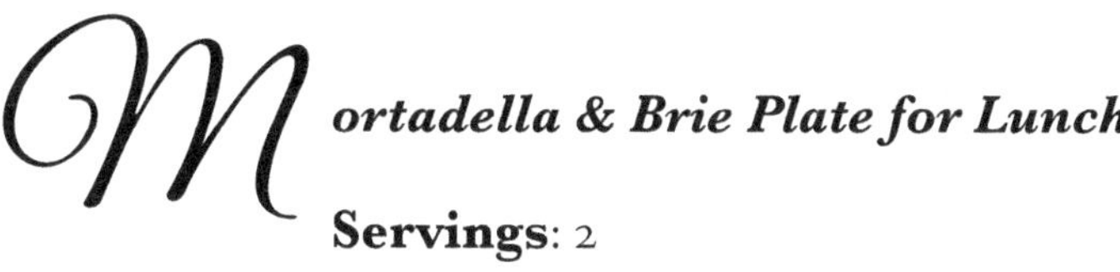

Mortadella & Brie Plate for Lunch

Servings: 2

Total Macros:

- 6 g Net Carbs
- 103 g Fat
- 40 g Protein
- 1118 Calories

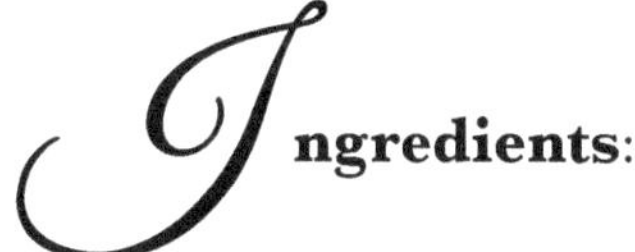

Ingredients:

- Italian mortadella sausage (9 oz.)
- Brie cheese or Camembert cheese (5 oz.)
- Anchovies (.66 oz.)
- Green pesto (2 tbsp.)
- Black olives (10)
- Arugula lettuce (6 oz.)
- Keto-friendly mayo (.5 cup)
- 10 leaves of fresh basil (10)

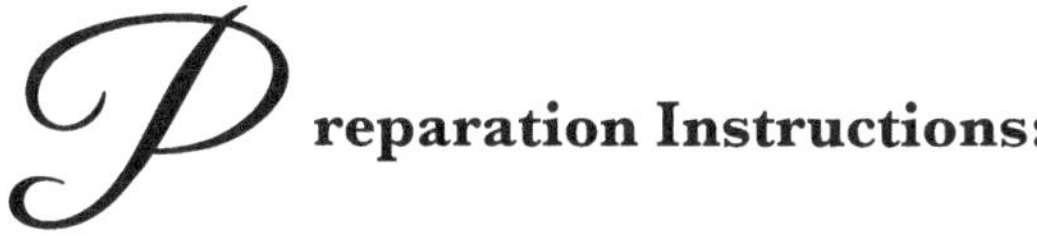

Preparation Instructions:

1. Arrange the thinly sliced mortadella, the anchovies, cheese, olives, pesto, and keto-friendly mayo on a platter.

2. Serve with the arugula and fresh basil.
3. Note: Mortadella is a large sausage or lunch meat made from pork.

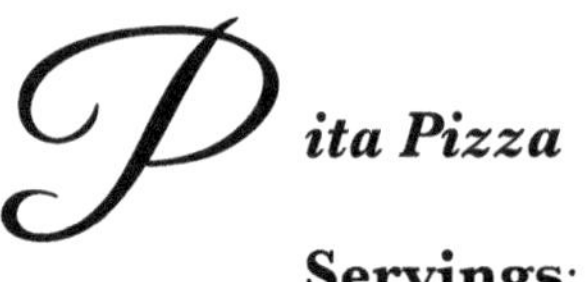

ita Pizza

Servings: 2

Total Macros:

- 4 g Net Carbs
- 19 g Fat
- 13 g Protein
- 250 Calories

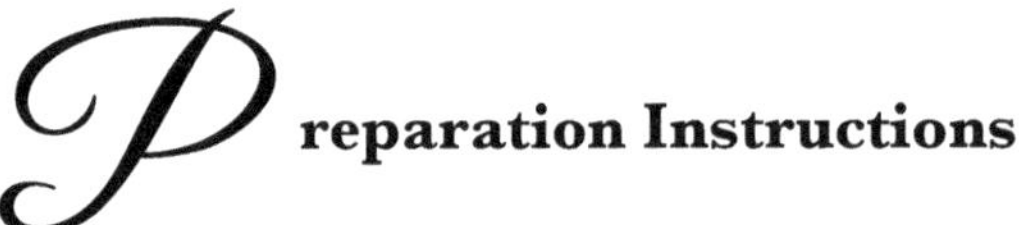

reparation Instructions:

- Marinara sauce (.5 cup)
- Low-carb pita (1)
- Cheddar cheese (2 oz.)
- Pepperoni (14 slices)
- Roasted red peppers (1 oz.)

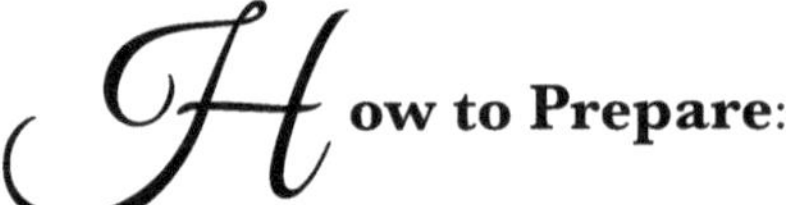

ow to Prepare:

1. Program the oven temperature setting to 450° Fahrenheit.
2. Slice the pita in half and place onto a foil-lined baking tray. Rub with a bit of oil and toast for one to two minutes.
3. Pour the sauce over the bread, sprinkle with the cheese, and other toppings. Bake for another five minutes or until the cheese melts.
4. Remove from the oven and let it cool thoroughly.

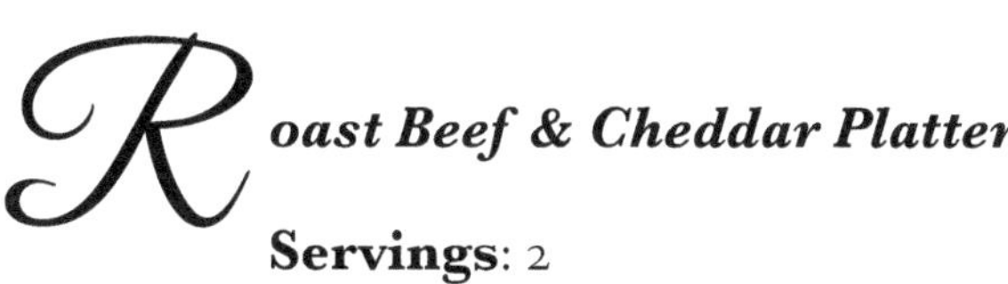

Roast Beef & Cheddar Platter

Servings: 2

Total Macros:

- 6 g Net Carbs
- 98 g Fat
- 38 g Protein
- 1072 Calories

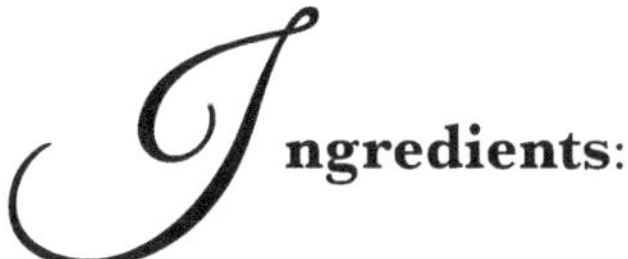

Ingredients:

- Deli roast beef (7 oz.)
- Cheddar cheese (5 oz.)
- Avocado (1)
- Radishes (6)

- Scallion (1)
- Mayonnaise (.5 cup)
- Dijon mustard (1 tbsp.)
- Lettuce (2 oz.)
- Olive oil (2 tbsp.)
- Pepper & Salt (as desired)

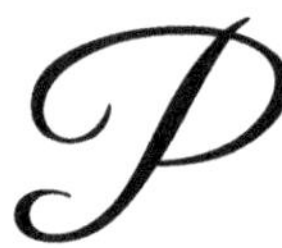

reparation Instructions:

1. Slice the onion.
2. Place the cheese, roast beef, radishes, and avocado on a serving platter.
3. Add the sliced onion, a dollop of mayo, and the mustard.
4. Serve with lettuce and a spritz of olive oil.

DINNER SPECIALTIES

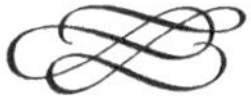

Beef Options

Pimiento Cheese Meatballs

Servings: 4

Total Macros:

- 1 g Net Carbs
- 53 g Fat
- 42 g Protein
- 660 Calories

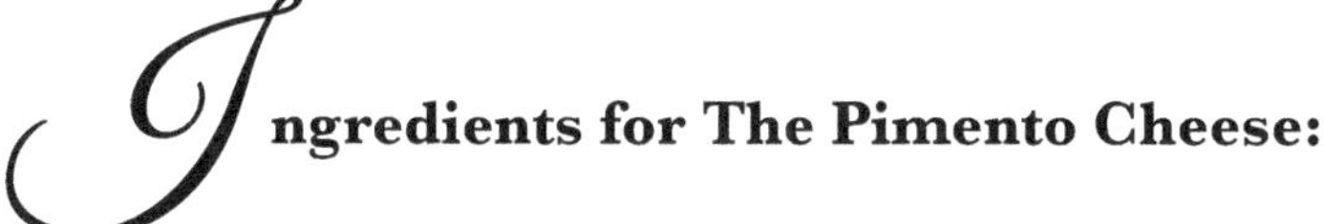

ngredients for The Pimento Cheese:

- Mayonnaise (.33 cup)
- Pimentos or pickled jalapeños (.25 cup)
- Paprika powder or chili powder (1 tsp.)
- Dijon mustard (1 tbsp.)
- Cayenne pepper (1 pinch)
- Grated cheddar cheese (4 oz.)

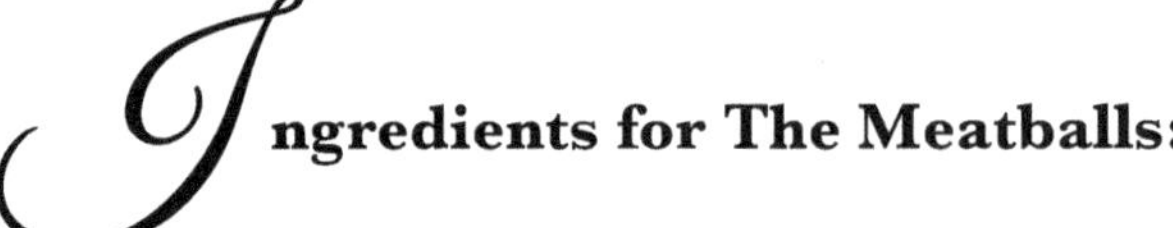

Ingredients for The Meatballs:

- Ground beef (.25 oz.)
- Egg (1)
- Salt and pepper
- Butter - for frying (2 tbsp.)

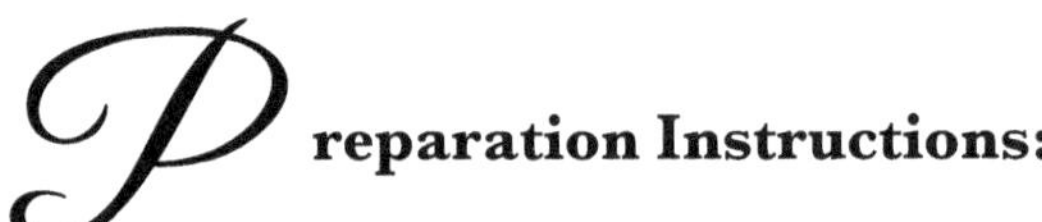

Preparation Instructions:

1. Prepare all of the ingredients for the cheese in a large mixing bowl and set aside for a few minutes.
2. Add the egg and the ground beef together and add to the rest of the ingredients. Sprinkle with the salt and pepper as desired.
3. Prepare the meatballs and fry them in oil or butter using the medium heat setting until they're done.
4. Serve with a salad of your choice.

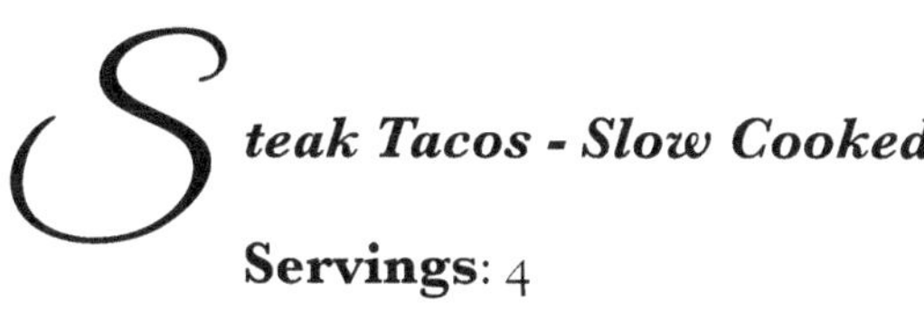

Steak Tacos - Slow Cooked

Servings: 4

Total Macros:

- 4 g Net Carbs
- 8 g Fat
- 25 g Protein
- 196 Calories

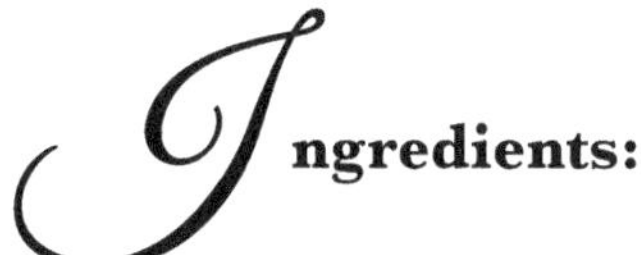

Ingredients:

- Chopped onion (.5 of 1)
- Bay leaves (1-2)
- Garlic cloves (4)
- Ancho chili powder (1.5 tsp.)
- Smoked paprika (1.5 tsp.)
- Salt & Ground black pepper (.5 tsp. each)
- Beef broth (.5 cup)
- Tri-tip roast (1 lb.)

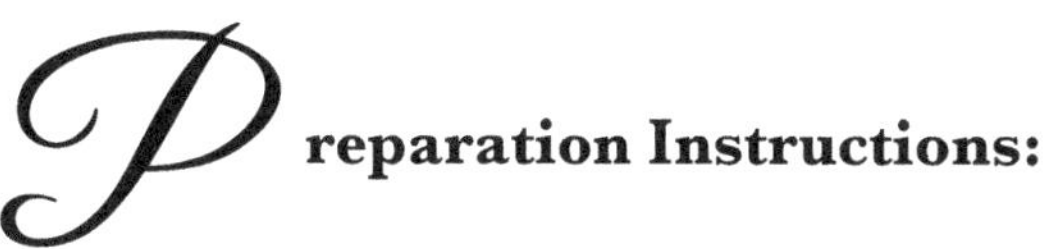

Preparation Instructions:

1. Remove the fat from the roast.
2. Mince the garlic into a paste using a garlic press or a food processor. You can also use the back of a knife and some coarse sea salt.
3. Combine the salt, pepper, chili powder, and paprika together to form a rub. Coat the meat.
4. Toss in the onions and empty the beef broth into the slow cooker, adding the meat last. Cook eight hours using the low setting.
5. Remove the lid and shred the meat about 30 minutes from the end of the cycle (7 ½ hrs.). Leave the cover off to simmer for the last 30 minutes.
6. Serve as a lettuce wrap or other favorite choice.

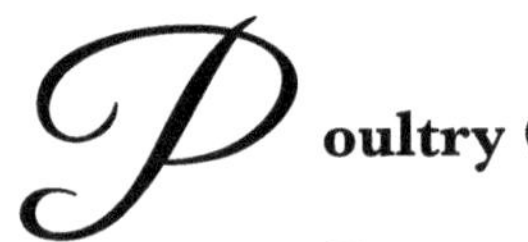

oultry Options

Fettuccine Chicken Alfredo

Servings: 2

Total Macros:

- 1 g Net Carbs
- 51 g Fat
- 25 g Protein
- 585 Calories

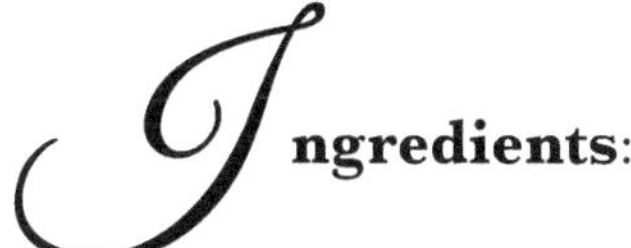

ngredients:

- Butter (2 tbsp.)
- Minced garlic cloves (2)
- Dried basil (.5 tsp.)
- Heavy cream (.5 cup)
- Grated parmesan (4 tbsp.)

Ingredients for The Chicken & Noodles

- Chicken thighs - no bones or skin (2)
- Olive oil (1 tbsp.)
- Miracle Noodle - Fettuccini (1 bag)
- Salt and pepper (as desired)

Preparation Instructions:

1. *For the Sauce*: Add the cloves to a pan with the butter for two minutes. Pour the cream into a skillet and let it simmer two additional minutes.
2. Toss in one tablespoon of the parmesan at a time. Add

the pepper, salt, and dried basil. Simmer 3-5 minutes on the low heat temperature setting.

3. *For the Chicken*: Pound the chicken with a meat tenderizer hammer until it's ½-inch thick. Warm up the oil in a skillet using the medium heat setting and put the chicken in to cook for about seven minutes per side. Shred and set aside.
4. *For the Noodles*: Prepare the package of noodles. Rinse, and boil them for two minutes in a pot of water.
5. Fold in the noodles along with the sauce and shredded chicken. Cook slowly for two minutes and serve.

Mozzarella & Pesto Chicken Casserole

Servings: 8

Total Macros:

- 3 g Net Carbs
- 30 g Fat
- 38 g Protein
- 451 Calories

Ingredients:

- Cooking oil (as needed)

- Grilled & cubed chicken breasts (2 lb.)
- Cream cheese (8 oz.)
- Cubed mozzarella (8 oz.)
- Shredded mozzarella (8 oz.)
- Pesto (.25 cup)
- Heavy cream (.25 to .5 cup)

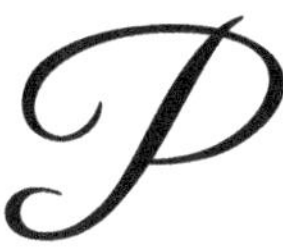**reparation Instructions**:

1. Warm up the oven to 400° Fahrenheit. Spritz a casserole dish with a spritz of cooking oil spray.
2. Combine the pesto, heavy cream, and softened cream cheese.
3. Add the chicken and cubed mozzarella into the greased dish.
4. Sprinkle the chicken using the mozzarella. Bake for 25-30 minutes.
5. Tip: Use 1/2 cup of cream if you prefer a thinner sauce or 1/4 cup for a thicker choice.

Nacho Chicken Casserole

Servings: 6

Total Macros:

- 4.3 g Net Carbs
- 32.2 g Fat
- 30.8 g Protein
- 426 Calories

Ingredients:

- Jalapeno pepper (1 medium)
- Chicken thighs (1.75 lb.)
- Pepper and salt (to taste)
- Olive oil (2 tbsp.)
- Chili seasoning (1.5 tsp.)
- Cheddar cheese (4 oz.)
- Cream cheese (4 oz.)
- Parmesan cheese (3 tbsp.)
- Green chilies and tomatoes (1 cup)
- Sour cream (.25 cup)
- Frozen cauliflower (1 pkg.)
- Also Needed: Immersion blender

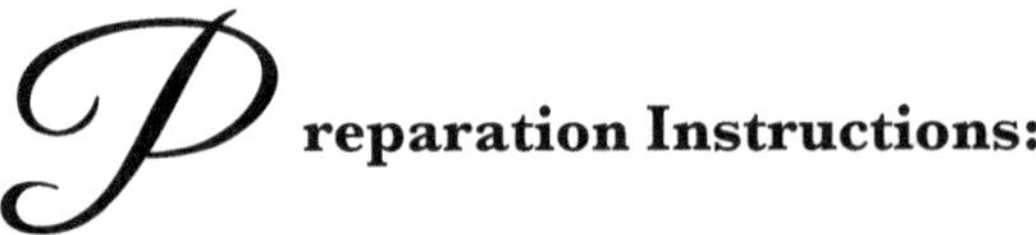

Preparation Instructions:

1. Heat up the oven to reach 375° Fahrenheit.
2. Slice the jalapeno into pieces and set aside.

3. Cut away the skin and bones from the chicken. Chop it up and sprinkle with the pepper and salt. Cook in olive oil using the medium-high temperature setting until browned.
4. Blend in the sour cream, cream cheese, and ¾ of the cheddar cheese. Stir until melted and combined well. Pour in the tomatoes and chilies. Stir and add it all to a baking dish.
5. Cook the cauliflower in the microwave. Blend in the rest of the cheese with the immersion blender until it resembles mashed potatoes. Season as desired.
6. Spread the cauliflower concoction over the casserole and sprinkle with the peppers. Bake approximately 15-20 minutes.

Pork & Lamb Options

Jamaican Jerk Pork Roast

Servings: 12

Total Macros:

- -0- g Net Carbs
- 20 g Fat
- 23 g Protein
- 282 Calories

Ingredients:

- Olive oil (1 tbsp.)
- Pork shoulder (4 lb.)
- Broth or beef stock (.5 cup)
- Jamaican Jerk spice blend (.25 cup)
- Also Needed: Dutch oven

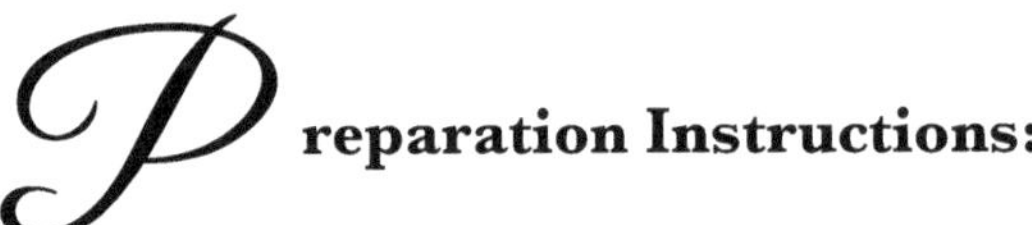

Preparation Instructions:

1. Rub the roast well the oil and coat with the jerk spice blend.
2. Use the Dutch oven to sear the roast on all sides. Add the beef broth.
3. Cover the pot and simmer for about four hours using the low heat setting. (You can also bake it for three hours at 375° Fahrenheit.)
4. Shred and serve.

Keto Lamb Chops & Herb Butter

Servings: 4

Total Macros:

- 0.3 g Net Carbs
- 62 g Fat
- 43 g Protein
- 729 Calories

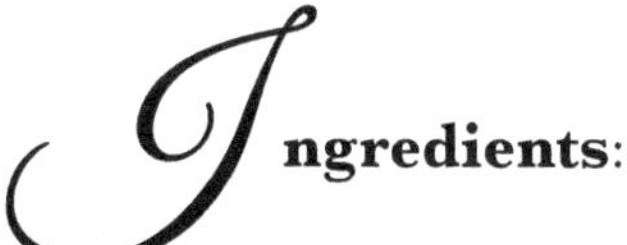

ngredients:

- Lamb chops (8)
- Pepper and salt (as desired)
- Olive oil (1 tbsp.)
- Butter (1 tbsp.)

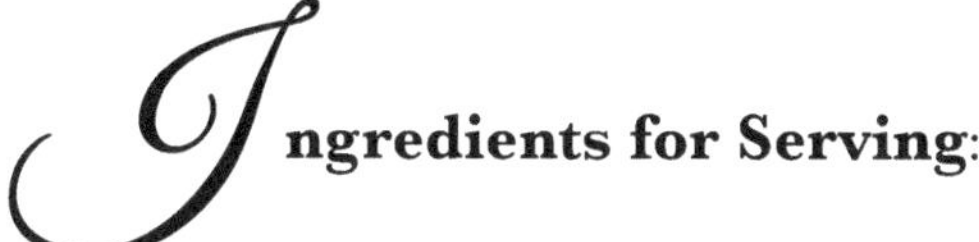

ngredients for Serving:

- Lemon (1)
- Herb butter (4 oz. - see recipe below)

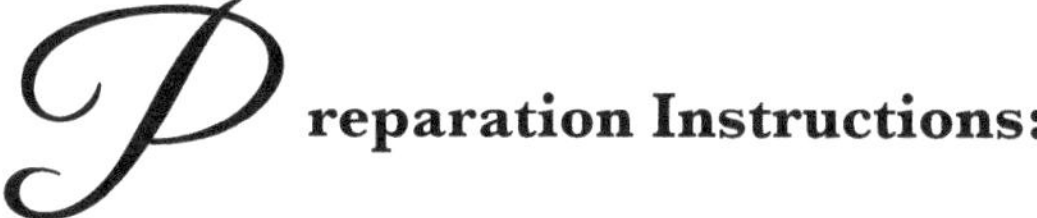

reparation Instructions:

1. Let the chops sit on the countertop until they become room temperature before you grill or fry them. Use a

sharp knife to make a few slashes in the fat part of the meat so it will not curl up.

2. Sprinkle with pepper and salt.
3. Add the oil and butter to a skillet or brush the grill with olive oil before adding the chops.
4. Fry for 3 to 4 minutes or until the lamb is a little bit pink inside.
5. Serve with herb butter and lemon wedges.

Keto Herb Butter

Servings: 4

Total Macros:

- 1 g Net Carbs
- 28 g Fat
- 1 g Protein
- 258 Calories

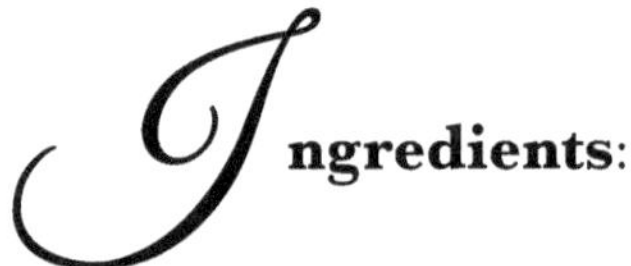

Ingredients:

- Butter, at room temperature (5 oz.)
- Pressed garlic clove (1)
- Garlic powder (.5 tbsp.)
- Finely chopped fresh parsley (4 tbsp.)
- Lemon juice (1 tsp.)

- Salt (.5 tsp.)

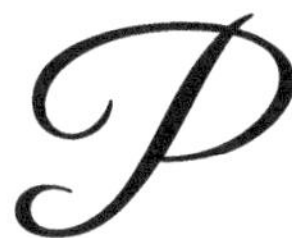

reparation Instructions:

1. Thoroughly mix the fixings in a mixing container. Set aside for about 15 minutes.
2. Store in the fridge until needed.

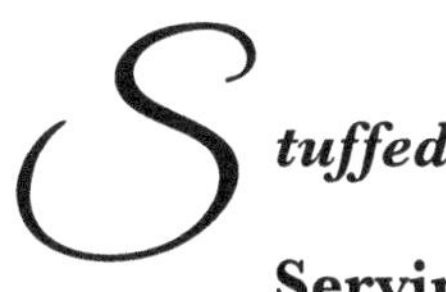

tuffed Pork Chops

Servings: 4

Total Macros:

- 1 g Net Carbs
- 38 g Fat
- 102 g Protein
- 778 Calories

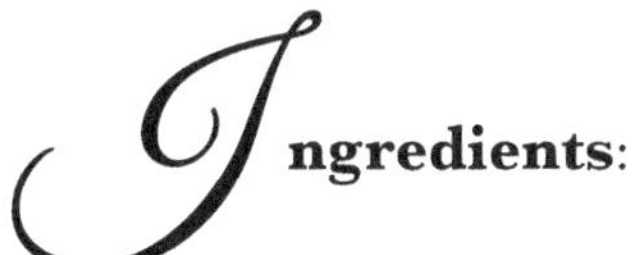

ngredients:

- Bacon (3 slices)
- Thick cut pork chops (4)

- Feta cheese (3 oz.)
- Blue cheese (3 oz.)
- Cream cheese (2 oz.)
- Green onion (.33 cup)
- Garlic powder (1 pinch)
- Black pepper & Salt (to your liking)

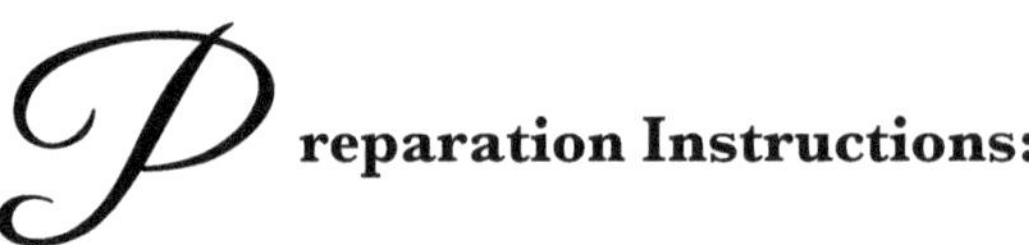

Preparation Instructions:

1. Program the oven temperature to 350° Fahrenheit. Lightly grease a baking tin.
2. Cook the bacon, reserving the grease and set aside.
3. Mix the feta and blue cheese. Blend in the onions and bacon. Next, add the cream cheese, and mix well.
4. Split the non-fat side of the pork and add the cheese mixture – closing with a toothpick. Sprinkle with the garlic powder, salt, and pepper.
5. Sear with the bacon grease in the skillet for 1.5 minutes per side.
6. Arrange the chops on the baking pan and cook for 55 minutes.
7. Let the chops rest about three minutes.

Fish Options

Beetroot-Cured Salmon with Dill Oil

Servings: 4

Total Macros:

- 4 g Net Carbs
- 42 g Fat
- 25 g Protein
- 500 Calories

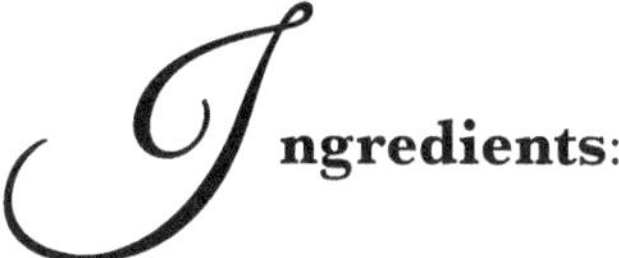

ngredients:

- Beet (1)
- Salt (2 tbsp.)
- White peppercorns (5)
- Lime - zested (1)
- Salmon (1 lb.)

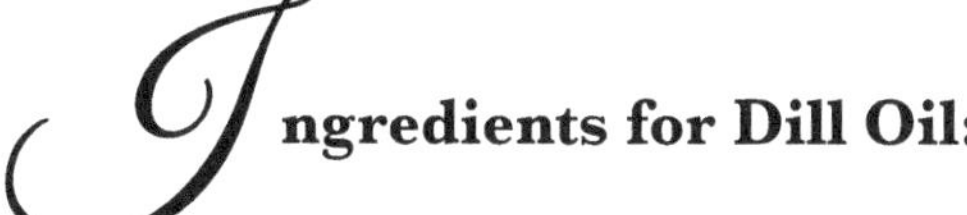

ngredients for Dill Oil:

- Chopped fresh dill (.5 cup)
- Frozen spinach (1 tbsp.)
- Light olive oil or avocado oil (.5 cup)
- Salt and pepper (to your liking)

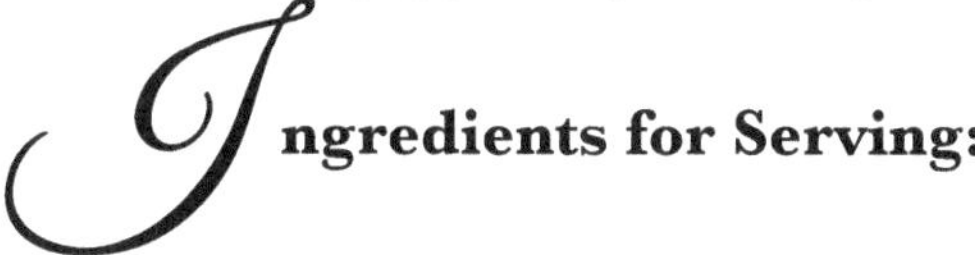

ngredients for Serving:

- Daikon - finely sliced (2 oz.)

- Lettuce (.5 lb.)

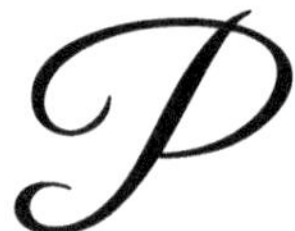

reparation Instructions:

1. Rinse the beetroot thoroughly and peel. Grate it coarsely and add it to a bowl along with the salt, peppercorn, and lime zest.
2. Partially defrost the salmon before the curing process.
3. Arrange the salmon with the skin side down and rub the flesh side evenly through the beetroot mixture. (You should probably wear a pair of gloves on your hands to prevent staining.)
4. Arrange the salmon in a glass dish with a piece of film over the top of it. Let it marinate in the fridge for one to two days, flipping halfway through the process.
5. Combine the spinach and dill with a hand blender. Mix in the oil, salt, and pepper.
6. Unwrap the salmon and brush off the beetroot cure (don't serve the marinade).
7. Cut the fish into thin slices and serve with the dill oil, chopped bacon, and leafy greens.

Lemon Garlic Shrimp Pasta

Servings: 4

Total Macros:

- 3.5 g Net Carbs

- 21 g Fat
- 36 g Protein
- 360 Calories

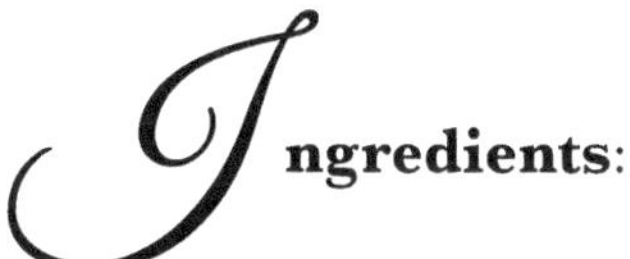

Ingredients:

- Angel hair pasta (2 bags)
- Garlic cloves (4)
- Olive oil (2 tbsp.)
- Butter (2 tbsp.)
- Lemon (.5 of 1)
- Large raw shrimp (1 lb.)
- Paprika (.5 tsp.)
- Fresh basil (as desired)
- Pepper and salt (to taste)

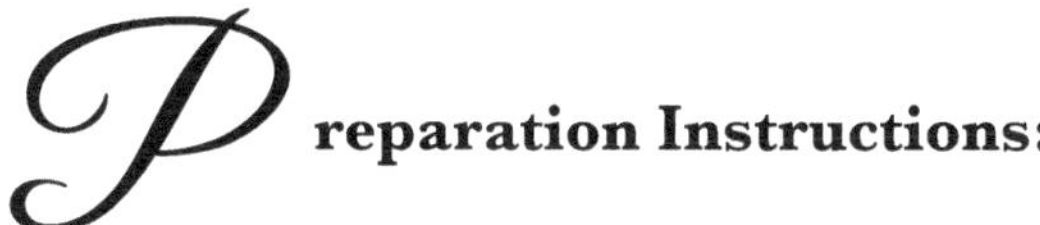

Preparation Instructions:

1. Drain the water from the package of noodles and rinse them in cold water. Add them to a pot of boiling water for two minutes. Transfer to a hot skillet over medium heat to remove the excess liquid (dry roast). Set them aside.
2. Use the same pan to warm the butter, oil, and mashed

garlic. Sauté a few minutes but *don't* brown.

3. Slice the lemon into rounds and add them to the garlic along with the shrimp. Sauté for approximately three minutes per side.
4. Add the noodles and spices and stir to blend the flavors.

KETO SNACK RECIPES

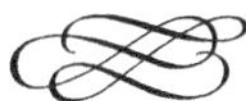

Blueberry Frozen Fat Bombs

Servings: 24

Total Macros:

- 1.02 g Net Carbs
- 13 g Fat
- .44 g Protein
- 116 Calories

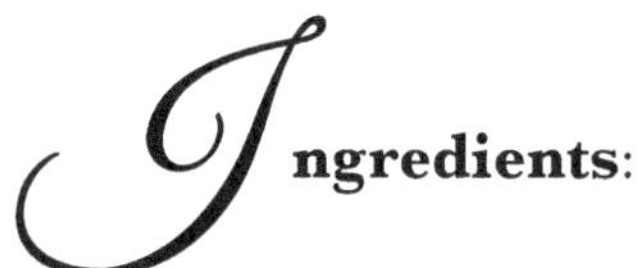

ngredients:

- Scant blueberries (1 cup)

- Coconut oil (.75 cup)
- Butter (1 stick)
- Coconut cream (.25 cup)
- Softened cream cheese (4 oz.)
- Sweetener of choice

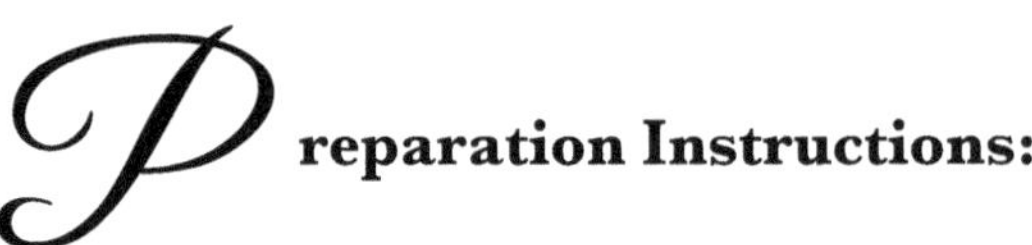

Preparation Instructions:

1. Arrange three to four berries in each mold cup.
2. Melt the coconut oil and butter over the lowest stovetop heat setting. Cool slightly for approximately five minutes.
3. Combine all of the ingredients and whisk well. Slowly, add the sweetener.
4. Using a spouted pitcher, fill an ice tray with 24 bombs.
5. Pop them out and eat when hunger strikes.

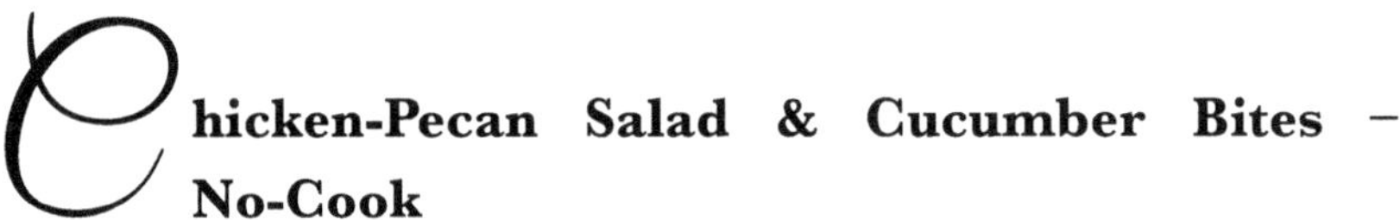

Chicken-Pecan Salad & Cucumber Bites – No-Cook

Servings: 2

Total Macros:

- 3 g Net Carbs
- 24 g Fat
- 23 g Protein
- 323 Calories

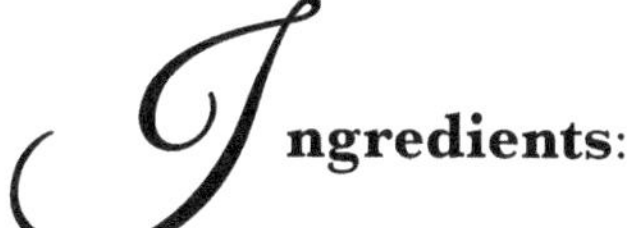

ngredients:

- Cucumber (1)
- Precooked chicken breast (1 cup)
- Diced celery (.25 cup)
- Mayonnaise (2 tbsp.)
- Chopped pecans (.25 cup)
- Pink salt – Himalayan & Black pepper (1 pinch of ea.)

Preparation Instructions:

1. Peel and slice the cucumber into 1/4-inch slices. Dice the chicken and celery. Chop the pecans. Combine the pecans, chicken, mayonnaise, and celery in a salad bowl. Sprinkle with the pepper and salt.
2. Lay out the cucumber slices and add a pinch of salt. Layer each one with a spoonful of the chicken salad. Serve.

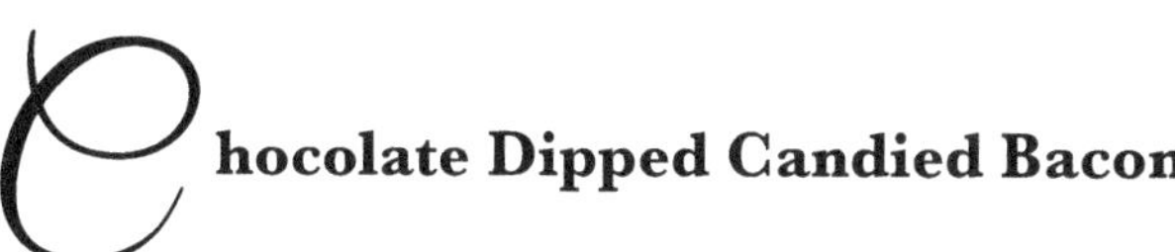

hocolate Dipped Candied Bacon

Servings: 16

Total Macros:

- 1.1 g Net Carbs
- 4.1 g Fat

- 3 g Protein
- 54 Calories

Ingredients:

- Thin-cut slices of bacon (16)
- Brown sugar alternative – ex. Surkin Gold or erythritol (2 tbsp.)
- Cinnamon (.5 tsp.)
- Cacao butter (.5 oz.) or coconut oil (1 tbsp.)
- 85% dark chocolate (3 oz.)
- Sugar-free maple extract (1 tsp.)

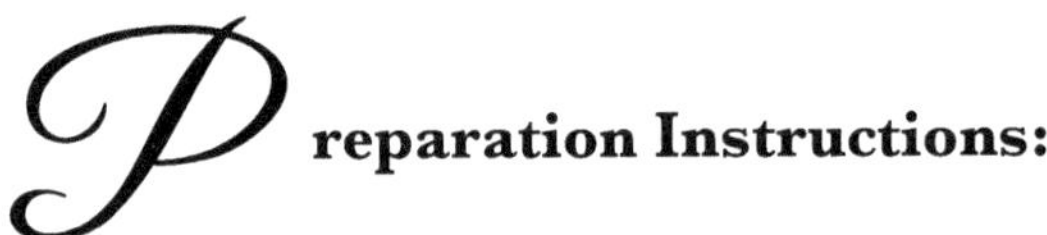

Preparation Instructions:

1. Mix the Surkin Gold sweetener with the cinnamon.
2. Lay the strips of bacon onto a parchment paper-lined tray. Sprinkle with 1/2 of the mixture.
3. Turn them over and do the other side with the rest of the mix.
4. Heat up the oven to reach 275° Fahrenheit. Bake until caramelized and crispy (60 to 75 min.).
5. Warm up a pan to melt the cocoa butter and chocolate.

Pour in the maple syrup and stir well. Set to the side until it's room temperature.

6. Arrange the bacon on a platter to cool thoroughly before dipping into the chocolate.
7. Dip 1/2 of each strip of the bacon in the chocolate. Place on a tray for the chocolate to solidify. You can place it in the fridge or just on the countertop.

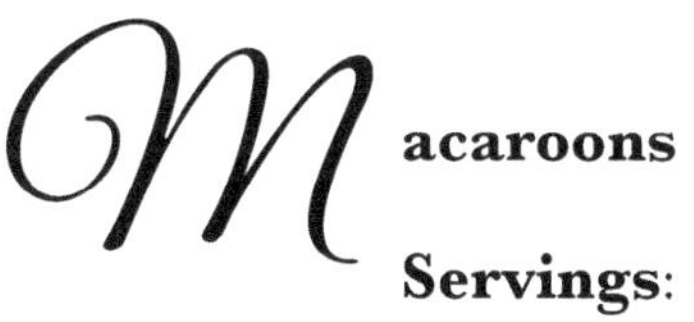

acaroons

Servings: 1

Total Macros:

- 4 g Net Carbs
- 10 g Fat
- 2 g Protein
- 90 Calories

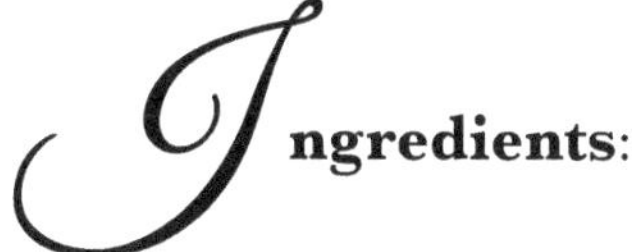

ngredients:

- Egg whites (4)
- Vanilla (1 tsp.)
- Artificial sweetener of choice (1 cup)
- Water (4.5 tsp.)
- Unsweetened coconut (.5 cup)

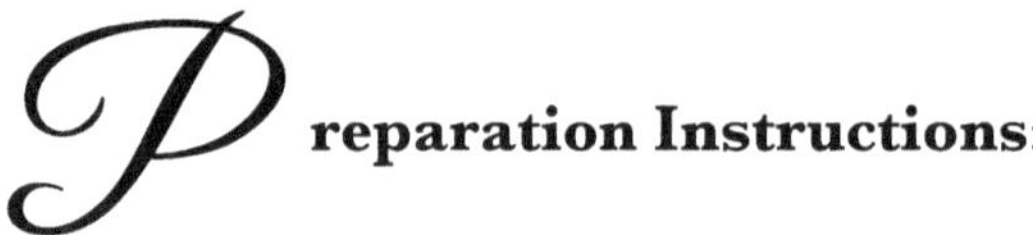

Preparation Instructions:

1. Heat up the oven to 325° Fahrenheit.
2. Whisk the eggs with the liquid components. Stir in the coconut and mix.
3. Use an immersion blender for uniform consistency.
4. Add the batter into the greased pan and bake for 15 minutes.

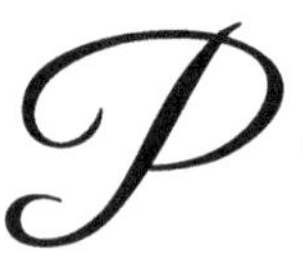

Peanut Butter & Coconut Balls

Servings: 15

Total Macros:

- 0.9 g Net Carbs
- 3.2 g Fat
- 0.98 g Protein
- 35 Calories

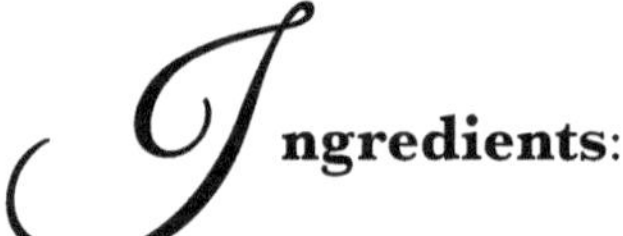

Ingredients:

- Powdered erythritol (2.5 tsp.)
- Creamy peanut butter – keto-friendly (3 tbsp.)

- Unsweetened cocoa powder (3 tsp.)
- Almond flour (2 tsp.)
- Unsweetened coconut flakes (.5 cup)

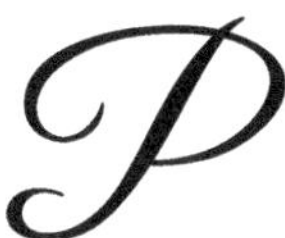

reparation Instructions:

1. Combine the peanut butter, cocoa, erythritol, and flour. Place in the freezer for one hour.
2. Spoon out a small spoon size of the peanut butter mix. Roll into the flakes until it is covered.
3. Refrigerate overnight for the best results.

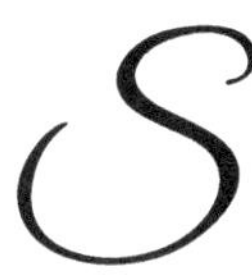

picy Deviled Eggs

Servings: 6

Total Macros:

- 1 g Net Carbs
- 19 g Fat
- 6 g Protein
- 200 Calories

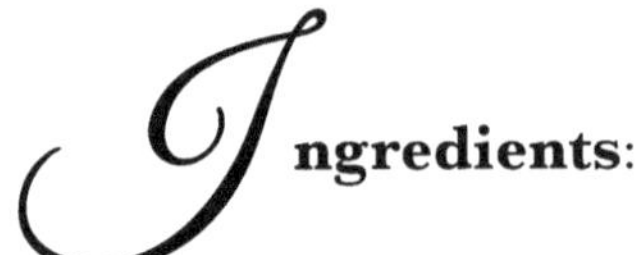

Ingredients:

- Eggs (6)
- Mayonnaise (.5 cup)
- Red curry paste (1 tbsp.)
- Poppy seeds (.5 tbsp.)
- Salt (.25 tsp.)

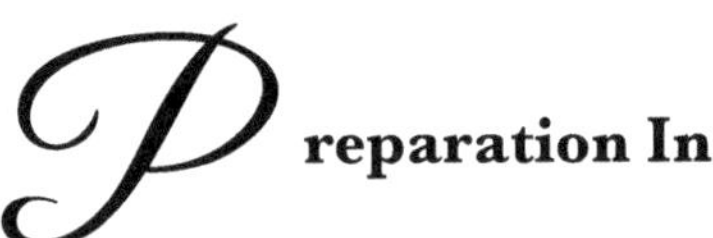

Preparation Instructions:

1. Prepare a pan with just enough water to cover the eggs. Do *not* put a lid on the pot but bring it to a boil.
2. Cook the eggs for about 8 minutes. Place into an ice water bath at that time.
3. Discard the egg shells and cut the eggs in half. Scoop out the egg yolk.
4. Place the whites on a platter and place it in the fridge.
5. Combine the mayonnaise, curry paste, and egg yolks until smooth.
6. Take the egg whites from the fridge and apply the prepared yolks. Sprinkle with the seeds on top to serve.

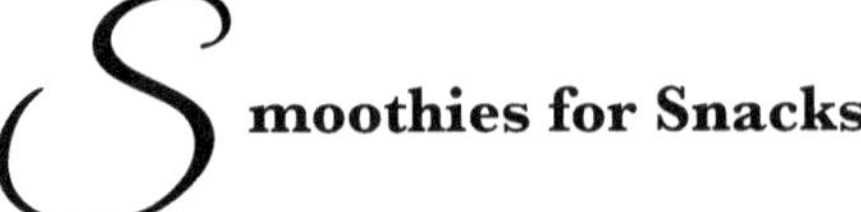

Smoothies for Snacks

Blueberry & Kefir Smoothie

Servings: 2

Total Macros:

- 6.6 g Net Carbs
- 50 g Fat
- 3.9 g Protein
- 476 Calories

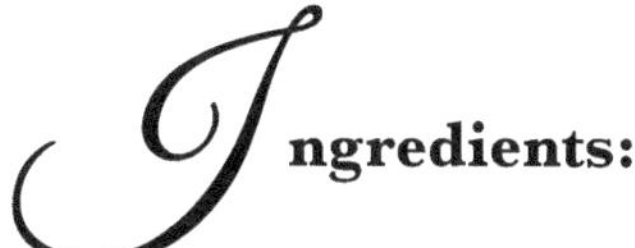

ngredients:

- Coconut milk kefir (1.5 cups)
- Fresh or frozen blueberries (.5 cup)
- MCT oil (2 tbsp.)
- Water (+) ice cubes (.5 cup)
- Sugar-free vanilla extract (1-2 tsp.) or pure vanilla powder (.5 tsp.)

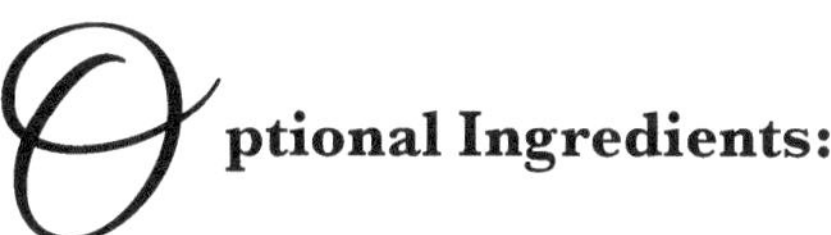

ptional Ingredients:

- Collagen powder (2 tbsp.)
- Drops liquid stevia/your choice (3-5 drops)

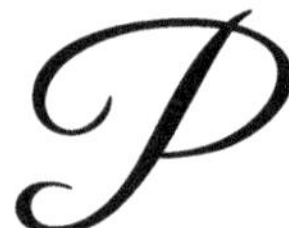

Preparation Instructions:

1. Toss all of the ingredients into your blender
2. Pulse until the fixings are well mixed.
3. Serve in chilled glasses.

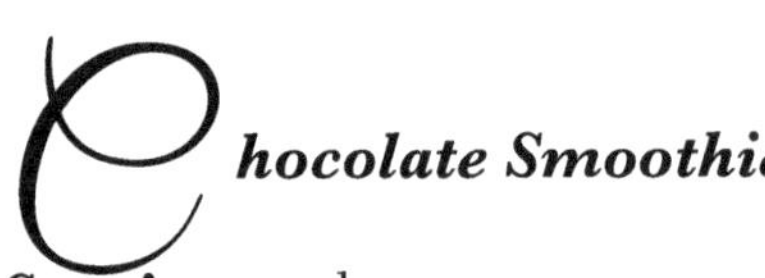

Chocolate Smoothie

Servings: 1 large

Total Macros:

- 4.4 g Net Carbs
- 46 g Fat
- 34.5 g Protein
- 570 Calories

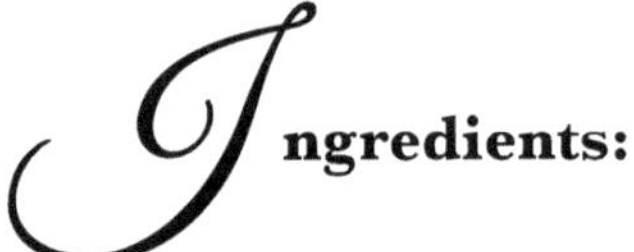

Ingredients:

- Large eggs (2)
- Almond or coconut butter (1-2 tbsp.)
- Extra-virgin coconut oil (1 tbsp.)
- Coconut milk or heavy whipping cream (.25 cup)
- Chia seeds (1-2 tbsp.)

- Cinnamon (.5 tsp.)
- Plain or chocolate whey protein (.25 cup)
- Stevia extract (3-5 drops)
- Unsweetened cacao powder (1 tbsp.)
- Water (.25 cup)
- Ice (.5 cup)
- Vanilla extract (.5 tsp.)

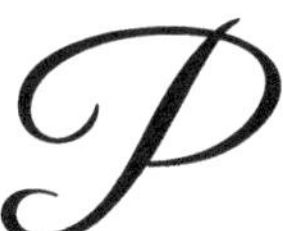 **reparation Instructions**:

1. Add the eggs along with the rest of fixings into the blender.
2. Pulse until frothy. Add to a chilled glass and enjoy.

Cinnamon Roll Smoothie

Servings: 1

Total Macros:

- 0.6 g Net Carbs
- 3.25 g Fat
- 26.5 g Protein
- 145 Calories

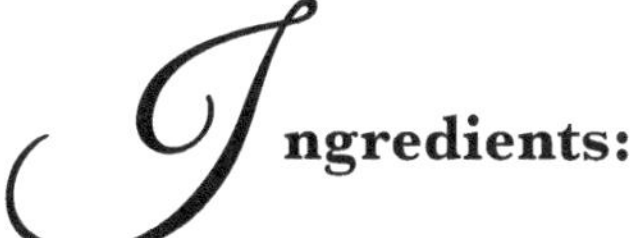 **ngredients:**

- Almond milk (1 cup)

- Vanilla protein powder (2 tbsp.)
- Vanilla extract (.25 tsp.)
- Cinnamon (.5 tsp.)
- Sweetener (4 tsp.)
- Flax meal (1 tsp.)
- Ice (1 cup)

Preparation Instructions:

1. Combine all of the fixings in a blender.
2. Add the ice last.
3. Blend on the high-speed setting for 30 seconds until thickened before serving.

Vanilla Fat-Burning Smoothie

Servings: 1

Total Macros:

- 4 g Net Carbs
- 64 g Fat
- 12 g Protein
- 651 Calories

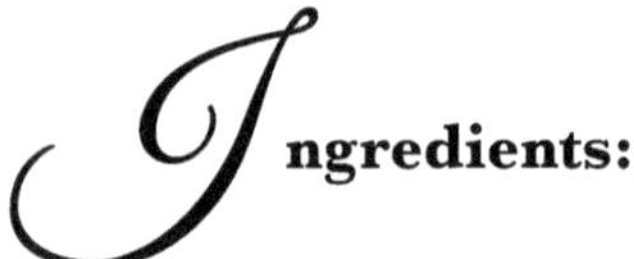

ngredients:

- Large egg yolks (2)
- Mascarpone full-fat cheese (.5 cup)

- Water (.25 cup)
- Coconut oil (1 tbsp.)
- Ice cubes (4)
- Liquid stevia (3 drops) or powdered erythritol (1 tbsp.)
- Pure vanilla extract (.5 tsp.)
- Optional topping: Whipped cream

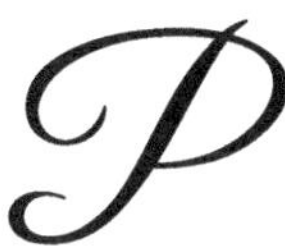

reparation Instructions:

1. Combine all of the fixings in a blender. Mix well.
2. Add the whipped cream for a special treat.

KETO DESSERT CHOICES

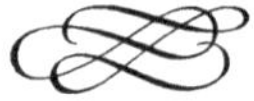

Chocolate Lava Cake

Servings: 4

Total Macros:

- 3 g Net Carbs
- 17 g Fat
- 8 g Protein
- 189 Calories

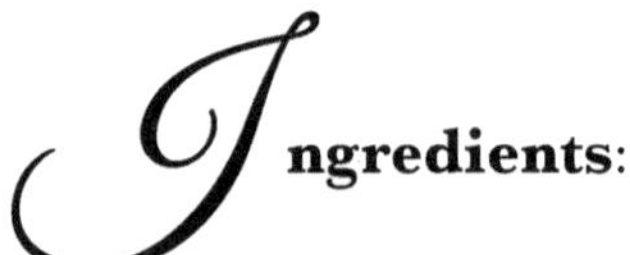**ngredients**:

- Unsweetened cocoa powder (.5 cup)
- Melted butter (.25 cup)

- Eggs (4)
- Sugar-free chocolate sauce (.25 cup)
- Sea salt (.5 tsp.)
- Ground cinnamon (.5 tsp.)
- Pure vanilla extract (1 tsp.)
- Stevia (.25 cup)
- Also Needed: Ice cube tray & 4 ramekins

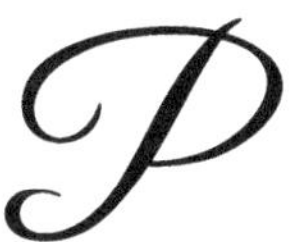

reparation Instructions:

1. Pour 1 tablespoon of the chocolate sauce into 4 of the tray slots and freeze.
2. Warm up the oven to 350° Fahrenheit. Lightly grease the ramekins with butter or a spritz of oil.
3. Mix the salt, cinnamon, cocoa powder, and stevia until combined. Whisk in the eggs – one at a time. Stir in the melted vanilla extract and butter.
4. Fill each of the ramekins halfway and add one of the frozen chocolates. Cover the rest of the container with the cake batter.
5. Bake for 13-14 minutes. When they're set, place on a wire rack to cool for about five minutes. Remove and put on a serving dish.
6. Enjoy by slicing its molten center.

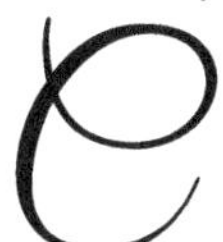

innamon Apple Muffins

Servings: 12

Total Macros:

- 3 g Net Carbs
- 22 g Fat
- 7 g Protein
- 241 Calories

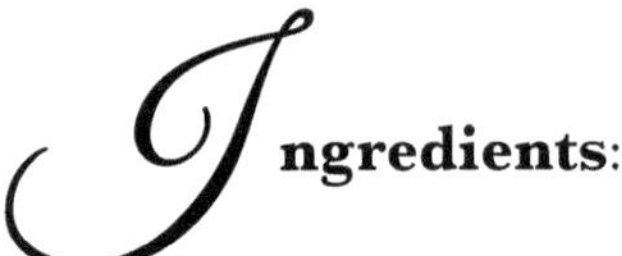

ngredients:

- Melted ghee (.5 cup)
- Large whisked eggs (3)
- Nutmeg (1 tsp.)
- Cinnamon (3 tbsp.)
- Almond flour (3 cups)
- Cloves (.25 tsp.)
- Applesauce (4 tbsp.)
- Baking powder (1 tsp.)
- Lemon juice (1 tsp.)
- Stevia (to your liking)
- Also Needed: 12-section muffin tins with paper or silicone cups

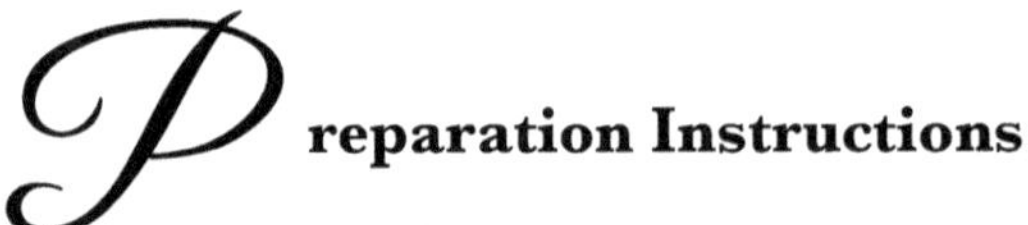

reparation Instructions:

1. Program the oven temperature setting to 350° Fahrenheit.

2. Combine the rest of the fixings in a mixing container.
3. Empty the batter into the prepared muffin tins.
4. Bake 17-20 minutes until the center is springy.

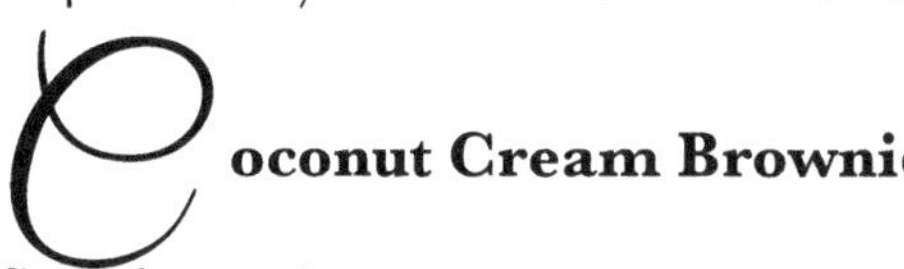

oconut Cream Brownies

Servings: 6

Total Macros:

- 2 g Net Carbs
- 17 g Fat
- 3 g Protein
- 175 Calories

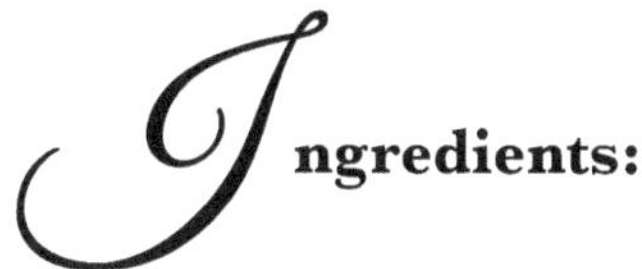

ngredients:

- Coconut cream (.33 cup)
- Melted coconut butter (.75 cup)
- Raw - unsweetened cocoa powder (.33 cup)
- Coconut flour (.33 cup)
- Melted butter or coconut oil (2 tbsp.)
- Stevia sugar substitute (.5 cup)
- Pure vanilla extract (1 tsp.)
- Sea salt (1 pinch)
- Egg (1)
- Baking soda (.25 tsp.)
- Also Needed: 3x9-inch loaf pan

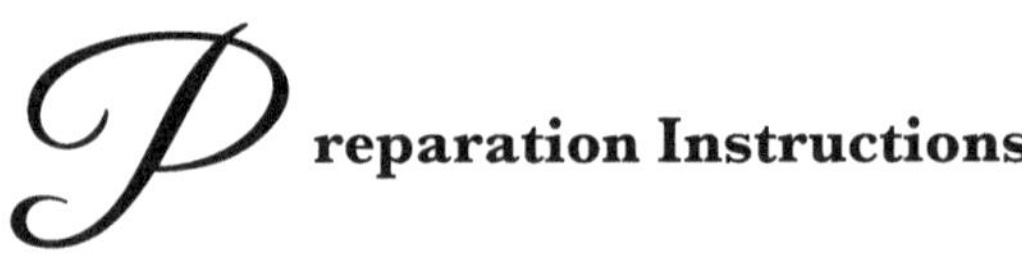

Preparation Instructions

1. Warm up the oven to reach 350° Fahrenheit.
2. Combine the stevia, salt, flour, cocoa powder, and baking powder.
3. Whisk the coconut cream and butter in another container. Once combined, mix in the vanilla and the whisked egg.
4. Combine all of the fixings well and add to the baking pan.
5. Bake for 20 minutes.
6. Once it's done, cool and slice into six equal squares.

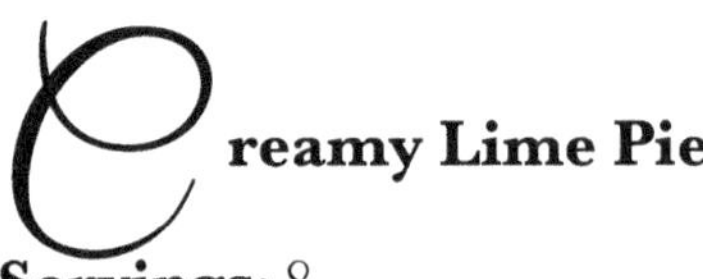

Creamy Lime Pie

Servings: 8

Total Macros:

- 4.2 g Net Carbs
- 39 g Fat
- 7 g Protein
- 386 Calories

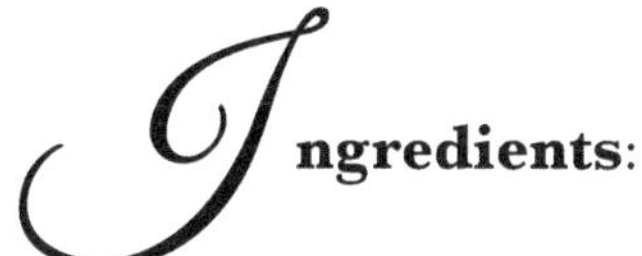

Ingredients:

- Almond flour (1.5 cups)
- Erythritol – divided (.5 cup)
- Salt (.5 tsp.)
- Melted butter (.25 cup)
- Heavy cream (1 cup)
- Egg yolks (4)
- Freshly squeezed key lime juice (.33 cup)
- Lime zest (1 tbsp.)
- Cubed cold butter (.25 cup)
- Vanilla extract (1 tsp.)
- Xanthan gum (.25 tsp.)
- Sour cream (1 cup)
- Cream cheese (.5 cup)

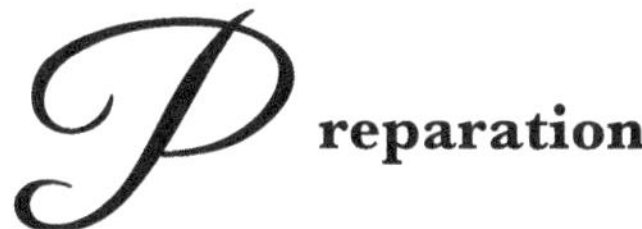

Preparation Instructions:

1. Warm up the oven to 350° Fahrenheit. Melt the butter in a pan.
2. Combine the salt, half or .25 cup of the erythritol, and the almond flour. Slowly add the butter. Blend and press into a pie platter.
3. Bake for 15 minutes. Remove when it's lightly browned. Let it cool.

4. In another saucepan, combine the egg yolks, heavy cream, rest of the erythritol, lime zest, and juice. Simmer over medium heat for 7 to 10 minutes or until it starts to thicken.
5. Take the pan from the heat. Stir in the xanthan gum, vanilla extract, cold butter, cream cheese, and sour cream. Whisk until smooth.
6. Scoop into the cooled pie shell.
7. Cover and place in the fridge for four hours. For best results, leave it overnight.

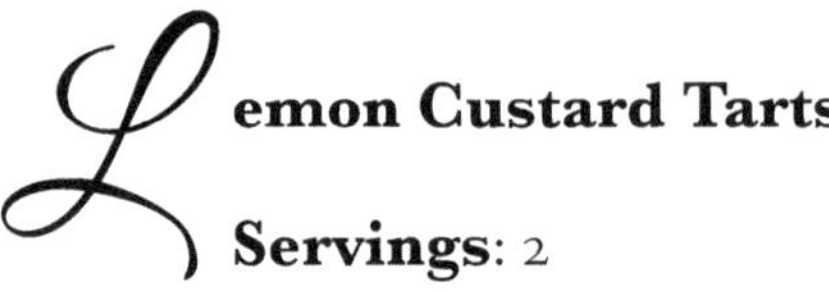

emon Custard Tarts

Servings: 2

Total Macros:

- 2 g Net Carbs
- 95 g Fat
- 17 g Protein
- 954 Calories

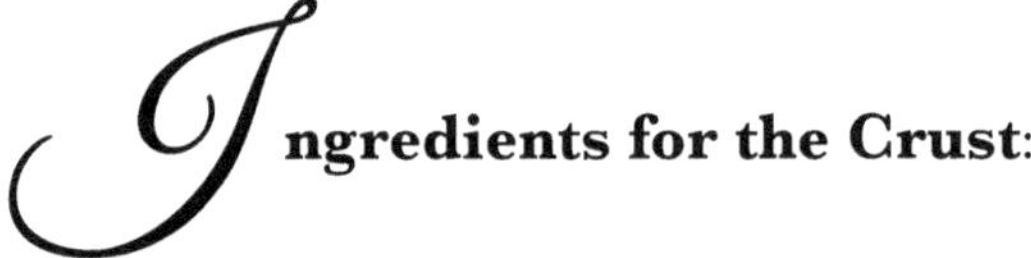

ngredients for the Crust:

- Unsalted melted butter (3 tbsp.)
- Almond meal (.75 cup)
- Optional: Dried lavender flowers (.5 tsp.)
- Sugar-free Vanilla bean sweetener syrup – ex. Torani (1 tbsp.)

Ingredients for The Filling:

- Freshly squeezed lemon juice (.5 cup)
- Large egg yolks (4)
- Grated zest of lemon (3)
- Unsalted butter – melted (.5 cup)
- Sugar-free vanilla syrup - your brand preference (.25 - .5 cup)
- Also Needed: 2 crème Brule dishes – 4.5-inch x 1.25 thick

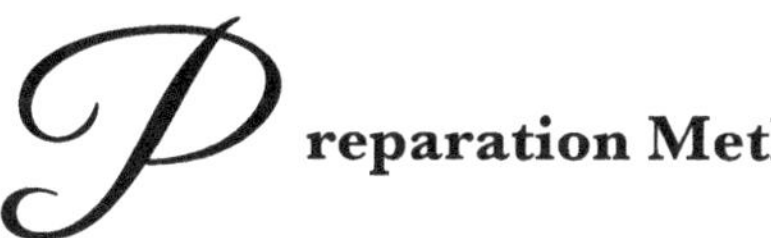

reparation Method:

1. Heat up the oven to 375° Fahrenheit.
2. Lightly spritz the dishes with some ghee or butter.
3. *Prepare the Crust*: If you're using the flowers, grind them into fine dust with a mortar and pestle. Combine with the 3 tablespoons of melted butter and almond flour. Press into the bottom of the two dishes.
4. Bake until the tops start browning (10 min.). Transfer to the counter to cool.
5. *Make the Filling*: Use a food processor or blender to mix the lemon juice, sweetener, egg yolks, lemon zest and rest

of the butter. Scoop into a saucepan (med-low) and simmer about 15 minutes or until it's pudding-like.

6. When ready, pour the filling over the two crusts. Secure a layer of plastic wrap over each one and refrigerate overnight.

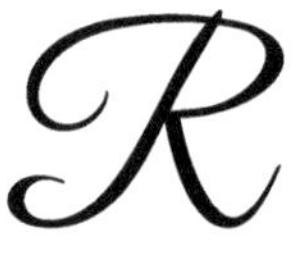

Raspberry Coconut Cake – Slow Cooker

Servings: 10

Total Macros:

- 7 g Net Carbs
- 32 g Fat
- 10 g Protein
- 362 Calories

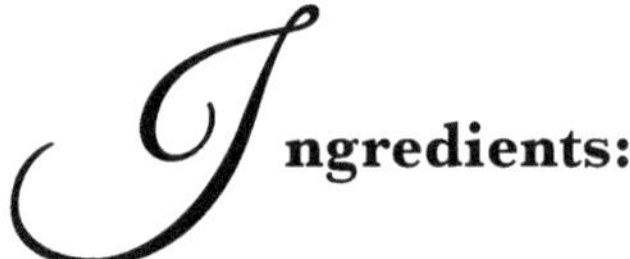

Ingredients:

- Unsweetened shredded coconut (1 cup)
- Almond flour (2 cups)
- Swerve sweetener (.75- 1 cup)
- Large eggs (4)
- Powdered egg whites (.25 cup)
- Salt (.25 tsp.)
- Baking soda (2 tsp.)
- Melted coconut oil (.5 cup)
- Raspberries – fresh or frozen (1 cup)
- Coconut extract (1 tsp.)

- Almond or coconut milk (.75 cup)
- Sugar-free dark chocolate chips (.33 cup)
- Coconut oil or favorite cooking spray
- Recommended: 6-quart size

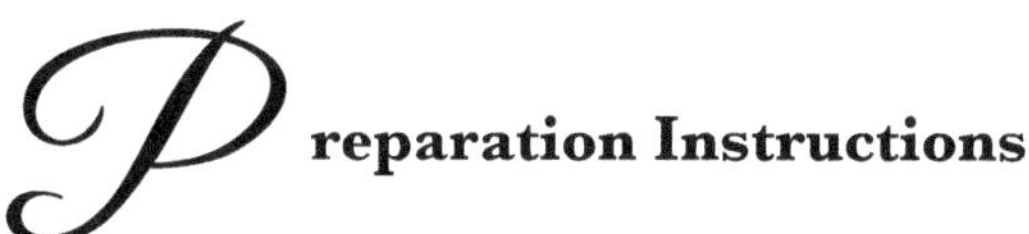

Preparation Instructions:

1. Spritz the inside of the cooker with cooking oil spray.
2. Whisk the flour, sweetener, coconut, salt, baking soda, and powdered egg whites in a large mixing container.
3. Add the coconut or almond milk, eggs, coconut extract, and melted coconut oil. Stir well and fold in the chips and berries.
4. Spread the prepared batter into the cooker and cook on the low setting for 3 hours. Turn the unit off and let it cool.
5. Top with whipped cream and serve.

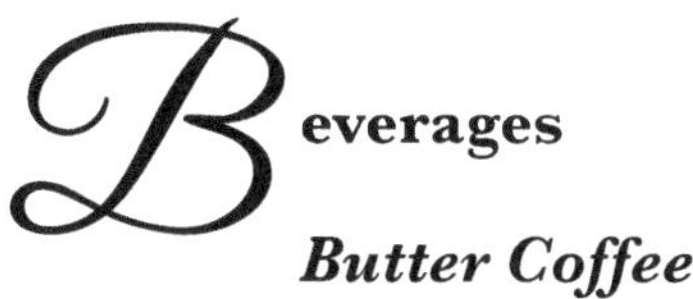

Beverages

Butter Coffee

Servings: 1

Total Macros:

- -0- g Net Carbs

- 25 g Fat
- -0- g Protein
- 230 Calories

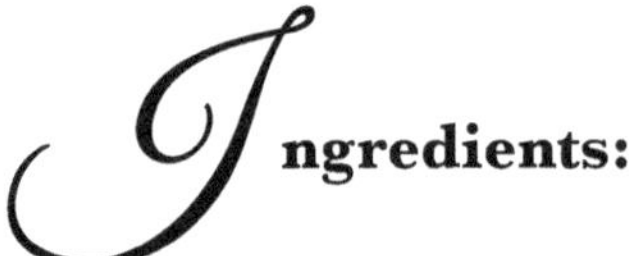

Ingredients:

- Coffee (2 tbsp.)
- Water (1 cup)
- Grass-fed butter (1 tbsp.)
- Coconut oil (1 tbsp.)

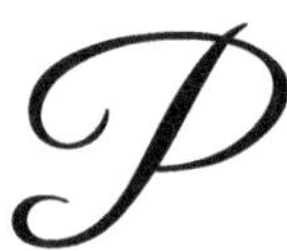

Preparation Instructions:

1. Prepare your favorite cup of coffee.
2. Combine the brewed coffee, butter, and coconut in a blender.
3. Puree about 10 seconds until it's light in color and creamy.
4. Enjoy anytime for a refreshing treat.

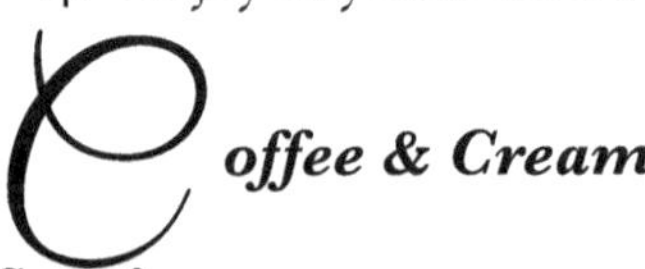

Coffee & Cream

Servings: 1

Total Macros:

- 2 g Net Carbs

- 22 g Fat
- 2 g Protein
- 206 Calories

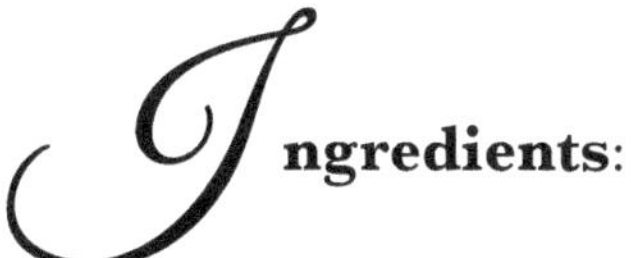

Ingredients:

- Coffee brewed to your liking (.75 cup)
- Heavy whipping cream (4 tbsp.)

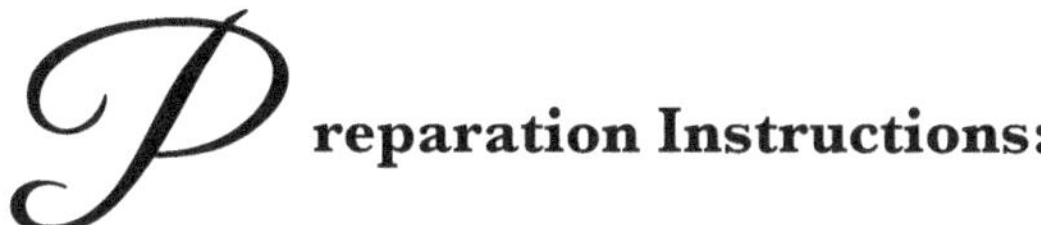

Preparation Instructions:

1. Prepare your coffee the way you want it.
2. Add the cream to a saucepan. Heat until it's frothy.
3. Pour the cream into a large mug, add the coffee, and stir.
4. Serve and enjoy with a slice of cheese and a handful of nuts for a snack or as it is.

Pumpkin Spice Latte

Servings: 1

Total Macros:

- 1 g Net Carbs
- 23 g Fat
- 0.5 g Protein
- 216 Calories

Ingredients:

- Unsalted butter (1 oz.)
- Instant coffee powder (1-2 tsp.)
- Pumpkin pie spice (1 tsp.)
- Boiling water (1 cup)

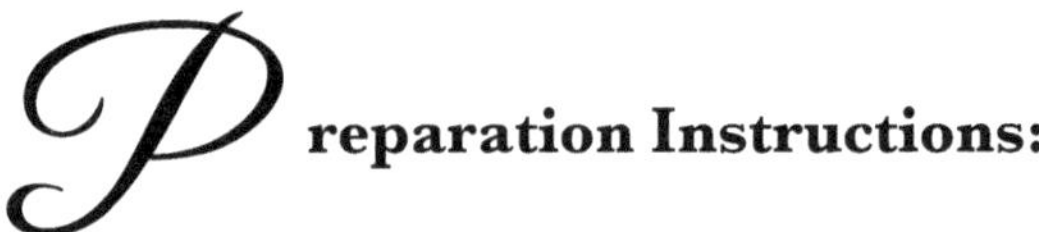

Preparation Instructions:

1. Use a deep container, and add the instant coffee, spices, and butter.
2. Blend using an immersion blender or add the fixings into the jar of a blender.
3. Add the water and blend another 20 to 30 seconds until it's foamy.
4. Pour into a mug and sprinkle with some pumpkin spice or cinnamon on top and serve. You can also add a dollop of whipped heavy cream.

15-DAY KETOGENIC DIET MEAL PLAN

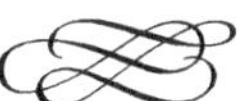

You can enjoy each of the recipes listed in your new meal plan since each one has the net carbs per serving posted. You will see how flexible the plan is when you look at how easy it is to use just the recipes in this cookbook for 15 full days including 3 meals, a snack, and dessert.

You can also enjoy other delicious tasty desserts and snacks at any time of the day or night. According to a favorite source: you should maintain the carb levels between 20 (optimal effect) to 50 net carbs daily.

Week One Recipes

Day 1: 21.2 Net Carbs

. . .

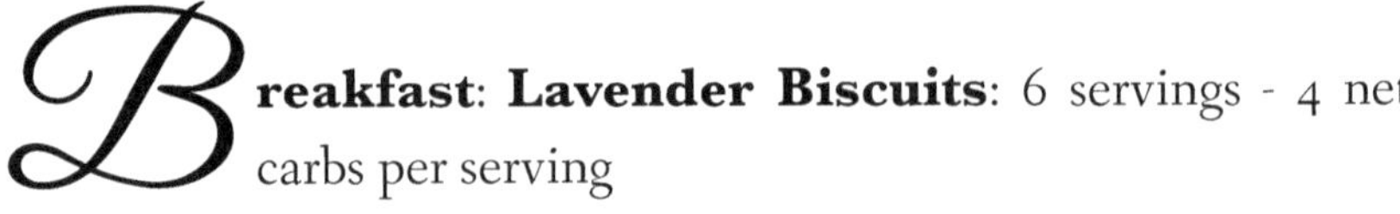

Breakfast: **Lavender Biscuits**: 6 servings - 4 net carbs per serving

Sausage Patties: 8 servings - 1.4 net carbs per serving

Snack: Cinnamon Roll Smoothie: 1 serving - 0.6 net carbs per serving

Lunch: **BLT In A Jar**: 8 servings - 7 net carbs per serving

Dinner: **Steak Tacos - Slow-Cooked**: 4 servings - 4 net carbs per serving

Dessert: **Creamy Lime Pie**: 8 servings - 4.2 net carbs per serving (leftovers)

Day 2: 18.5 Net Carbs

Breakfast: **Blueberry Ricotta Pancakes**: 5 servings - 6 net carbs per serving

. . .

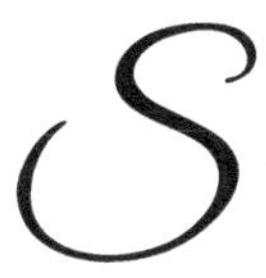**nack: Spicy Deviled Eggs**: 6 servings - 1 net carb per serving

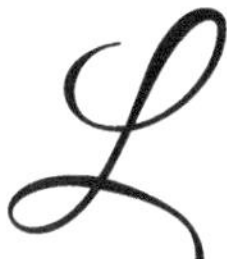**unch**: **Salad Sandwiches**: 1 serving - 3 net carbs per serving

**inner**: **Nacho Chicken Casserole**: 6 servings - 4.3 net carbs per serving

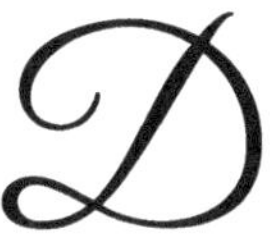**esert**: **Creamy Lime Pie**: 8 servings - 4.2 net carbs per serving

**ay 3: 14.1 Net Carbs**

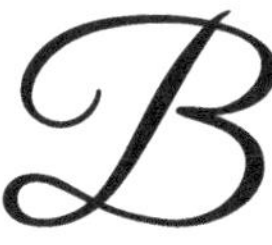**reakfast**: **Oven-Baked Pancake with Onions & Bacon**: 4 servings - 5 net carbs per serving

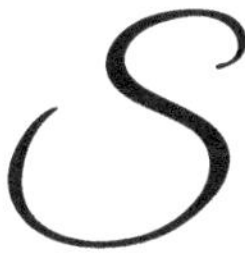**nack: Chocolate Dipped Candied Bacon**: 16 servings - 1.1 net carbs per serving

. . .

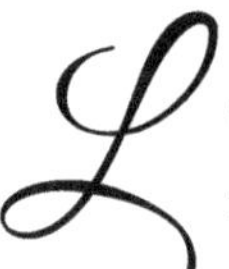unch: **Cauliflower & Citrus Salad**: 4 serving - 1 net carb per serving

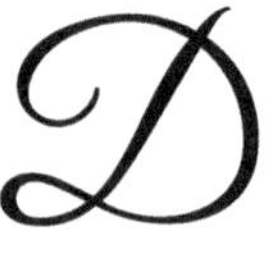**inner**: **Jamaican Jerk Pork Roast**: 12 servings - 0 net carbs per serving

with??

**essert**: **Raspberry Coconut Cake – Slow Cooker**: 10 servings - 7 net carbs per serving

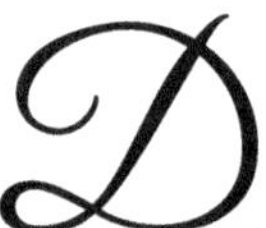**ay 4: 22 Net Carbs**

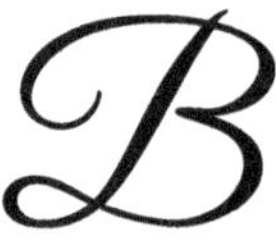**reakfast**: **Bacon & Cheese Frittata**: 6 servings - 2 net carbs per serving

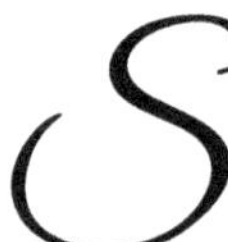**nack: Vanilla Fat-Burning Smoothie**: 1 serving - 4 net carbs per serving

**unch**: **Roast Beef & Cheddar Platter**: 2 servings - 6 net carbs per serving

. . .

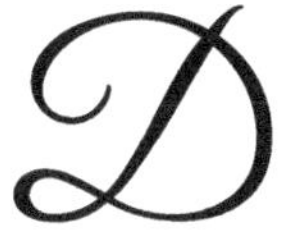inner: **Mozzarella & Pesto Chicken Casserole**: 8 servings - 3 net carbs per serving

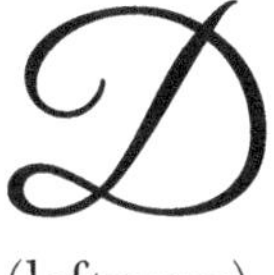essert: **Raspberry Coconut Cake – Slow Cooker**: 10 servings - 7 net carbs per serving (leftovers)

**ay 5: 16.02 Net Carbs**

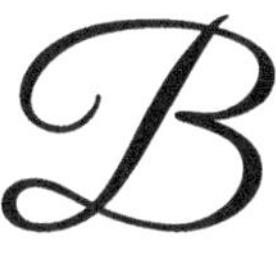**reakfast**: **Mushroom Omelet**: 1 serving - 4 net carbs per serving

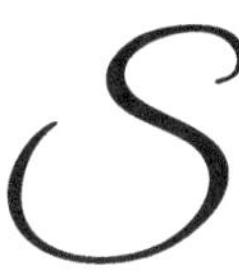**nack: Blueberry Frozen Fat Bombs**: 24 servings - 1.02 net carbs per serving

**unch**: **Cheeseburger Calzone**: 8 servings - 3 net carbs per serving

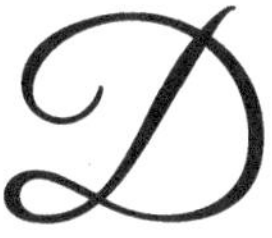**inner**: **Beetroot-Cured Salmon with Dill Oil**: 4 servings - 4 net carbs per serving

. . .

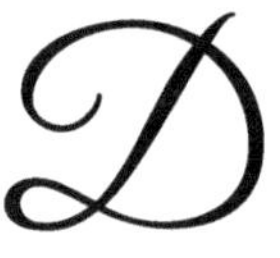essert: **Cinnamon Apple Muffins**: 12 servings - 3 net carbs per serving

**ay 6: 10.2 Net Carbs**

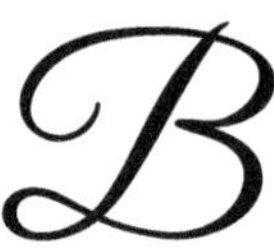**reakfast**: **Avocado & Bacon Omelet**: 1 serving - 3.3 net carbs per serving

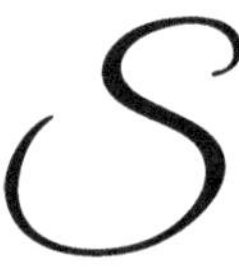**nack: Peanut Butter & Coconut Balls**: 15 servings - 0.9 net carbs per serving

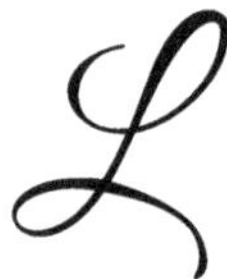**unch**: **Swedish Shrimp Salad with Dill**: 4 servings - 2 net carbs per serving

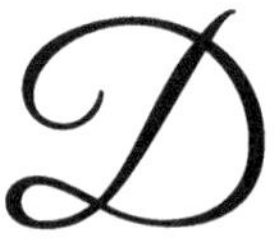**inner**: **Stuffed Pork Chops**: 4 servings - 1 net carb per serving

**essert**: **Cinnamon Apple Muffins**: 12 servings - 3 net carbs per serving

(leftovers)

. . .

**ay 7:** 20.02 Net Carbs

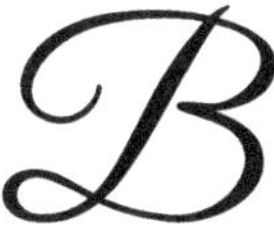**reakfast**: **Almost "McGriddle" Casserole**: 8 servings - 3 net carbs per serving

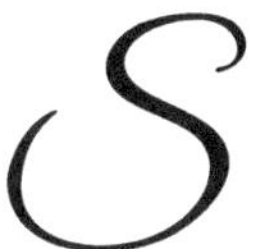**nack: Blueberry Frozen Fat Bombs**: 24 servings - 1.02 net carbs per serving

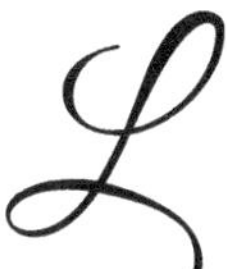**unch**: **Mortadella & Brie Plate for Lunch**: 2 servings - 6 net carbs per serving

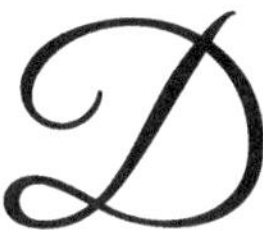**inner**: **Mozzarella & Pesto Chicken Casserole**: 8 servings - 3 net carbs per serving

**essert**: **Lemon Custard Tarts**: 2 servings - 2 net carbs per serving

Week Two Recipes

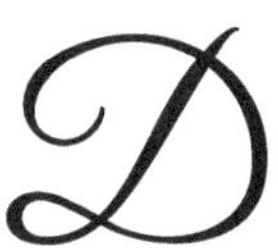**ay 8:** 15 Net Carbs

. . .

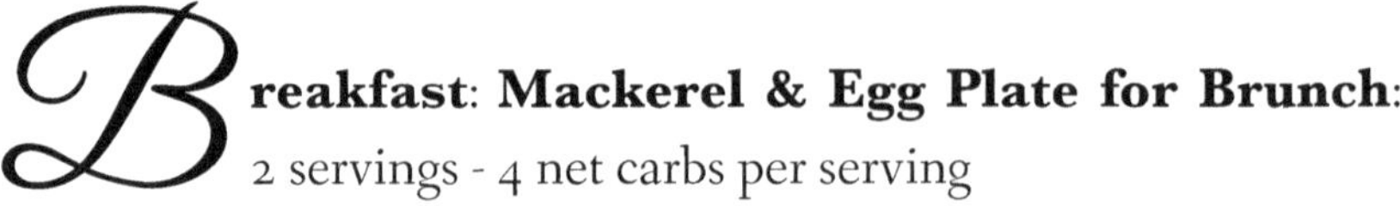

Breakfast: **Mackerel & Egg Plate for Brunch**: 2 servings - 4 net carbs per serving

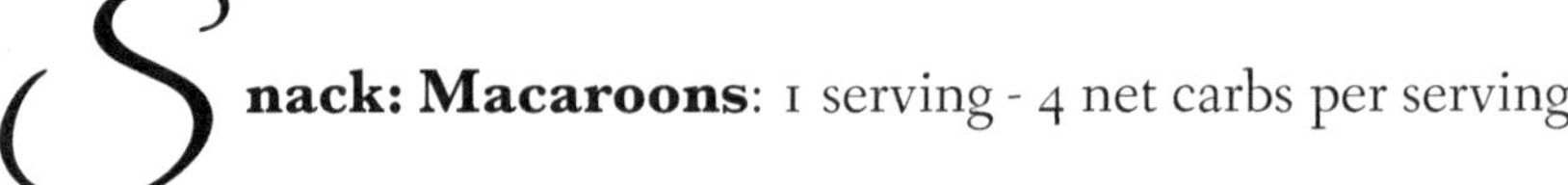

Snack: Macaroons: 1 serving - 4 net carbs per serving

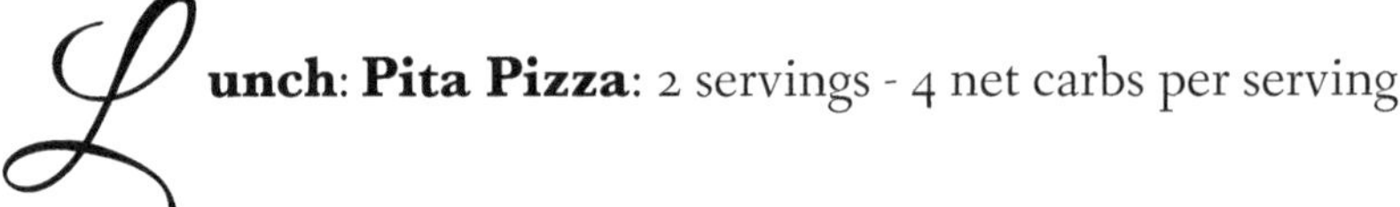

Lunch: **Pita Pizza**: 2 servings - 4 net carbs per serving

Dinner: **Jamaican Jerk Pork Roast**: 12 servings - 0 net carbs per serving

Dessert: **Chocolate Lava Cake**: 4 servings - 3 net carbs per serving

Day 9: 16.6 Net Carbs

Breakfast: **Blueberry & Kefir Smoothie**: 2 servings - 6.6 net carbs per serving

Snack: Chicken-Pecan Salad & Cucumber Bites – No-Cook: 2 servings - 3 net carbs per serving

. . .

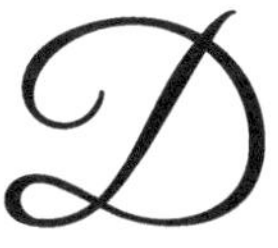**unch**: **Chicken "Zoodle" Soup**: 2 servings - 4 net carbs per serving

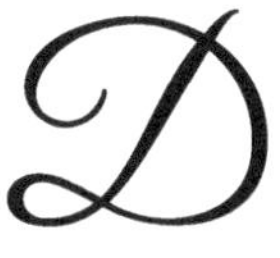**inner**: **Pimiento Cheese Meatballs**: 4 servings - 1 net carb per serving

**essert**: **Coconut Cream Brownies**: 6 servings - 2 net carbs per serving

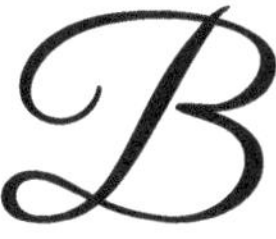**ay 10:** 16.4 Net Carbs

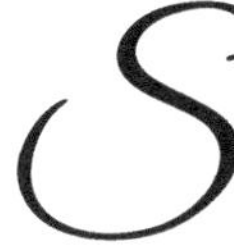**reakfast**: **Delicious Fully Herbed 'Fatty' Omelet**: 1 serving - 3.3 net carbs per serving

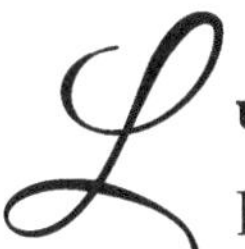**nack: Peanut Butter & Coconut Balls**: 15 servings - 0.9 net carbs per serving

unch: **Pork Lettuce Wraps**: 4 servings - 7 net carbs per serving

. . .

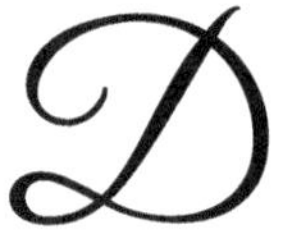**inner**: **Fettuccine Chicken Alfredo**: 2 servings - 1 net carb per serving

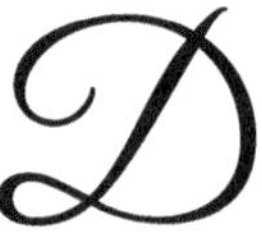**essert**: **Creamy Lime Pie**: 8 servings - 4.2 net carbs per serving

**ay 11:** 20.2 Net Carbs

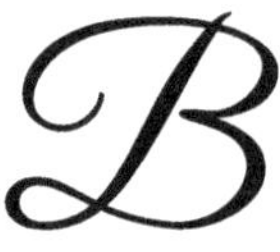**reakfast**: **Almost "McGriddle" Casserole**: 8 servings - 3 net carbs per serving

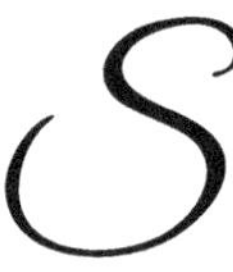**nack: Vanilla Fat-Burning Smoothie**: 1 serving - 4 net carbs per serving

Lunch: **Chicken Cakes**: 6 servings - 3.7 net carbs per serving

Lavender Biscuits: 6 servings - 4 net carbs per serving

Dinner: **Keto Lamb Chops & Herb Butter**: 4 servings - 0.3 net carbs per serving - **Keto Herb Butter**: 4 servings - 1 net carb per serving

. . .

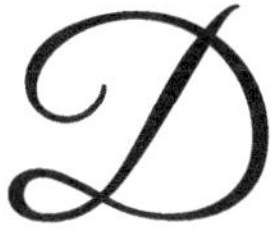essert: **Creamy Lime Pie**: 8 servings - 4.2 net carbs per serving

(leftovers)

**ay 12:** 19.5 Net Carbs

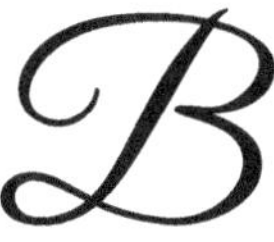**reakfast**: **Bacon & Cheese Frittata**: 6 servings - 2 net carbs per serving

**nack: Macaroons**: 1 serving - 4 net carbs per serving

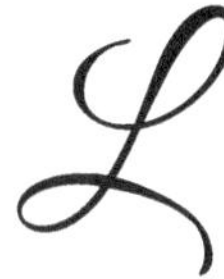**unch**: **Curry Chicken Lettuce Wraps**: 2 servings - 7 net carbs per serving

**inner**: **Lemon Garlic Shrimp Pasta**: 4 servings - 3.5 net carbs per serving

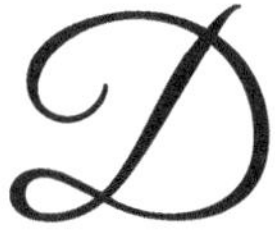**essert**: **Cinnamon Apple Muffins**: 12 servings - 3 net carbs per serving

. . .

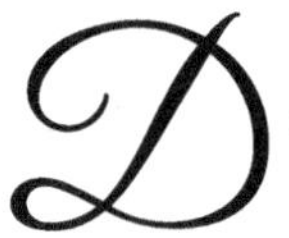**ay 13:** 12.4 Net Carbs

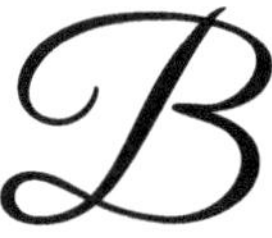**reakfast**: **Delicious Fully Herbed 'Fatty' Omelet**: 1 serving - 3.3 net carbs per serving

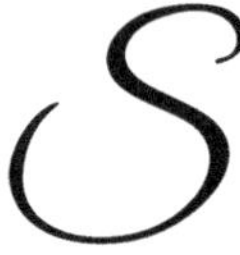**nack: Chocolate Dipped Candied Bacon**: 16 servings - 1.1 net carbs per serving

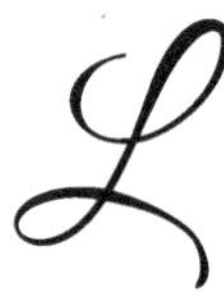**unch**: **Cauliflower & Citrus Salad**: 4 serving - 1 net carb per serving

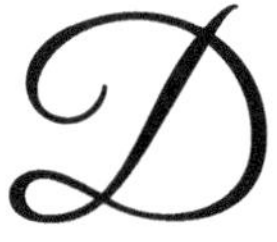**inner**: **Steak Tacos - Slow-Cooked**: 4 servings - 4 net carbs per serving

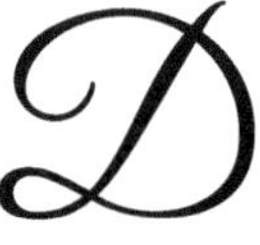**essert**: **Chocolate Lava Cake**: 4 servings - 3 net carbs per serving

**ay 14:** 13.6 Net Carbs

. . .

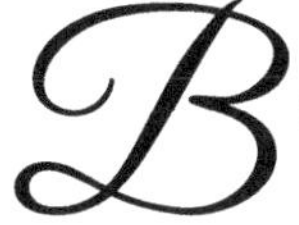**reakfast**: **Avocado & Bacon Omelet**: 1 serving - 3.3 net carbs per serving

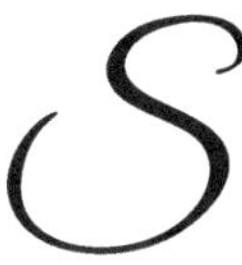**nack: Spicy Deviled Eggs**: 6 servings - 1 net carb per serving

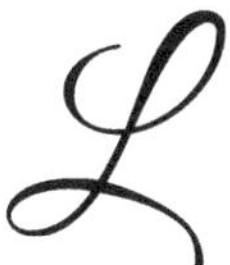**unch**: **Salad Sandwiches**: 1 serving - 3 net carbs per serving

**inner**: **Nacho Chicken Casserole**: 6 servings - 4.3 net carbs per serving

**essert**: **Lemon Custard Tarts**: 2 servings - 2 net carbs per serving

**ay 15:** 15.4 Net Carbs

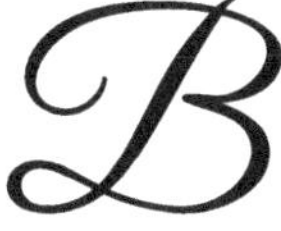**reakfast**: **Mushroom Omelet**: 1 serving - 4 net carbs per serving

. . .

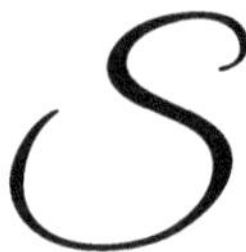**nack: Chocolate Smoothie:** 1 large serving: 4.4 net carbs per serving

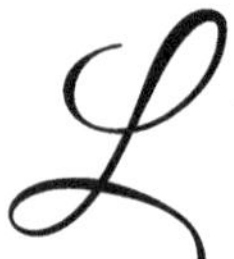**unch**: **Pita Pizza**: 2 servings - 4 net carbs per serving

**inner**: **Stuffed Pork Chops**: 4 servings - 1 net carb per serving

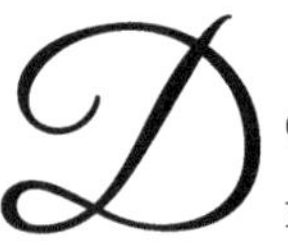**essert**: **Coconut Cream Brownies**: 6 servings - 2 net carbs per serving

You should have the basics of how to plan your meals using your new cookbook and guidelines. As you see, each of the recipes falls into the category of between 20 and 50 net carbs as used with the ketogenic diet plan. You can add to the meal plan according to the number of carbs you choose for your 'personal' plan.

CONCLUSION

I hope you better understand the ketogenic diet plan and the many ways it can be a part of your future. By reading the *Keto Diet for Beginners: Easy Everyday Low Carb Recipes – 15-Day Meal Plan,* you should have all of the tools you need to achieve your goals whatever they may be. The information provided will give you plenty of options for your new 15-Day meal plan.

At first, you may not notice the weight loss. There could be days or weeks where you don't see the changes, but slow is the best method. You are altering your lifestyle and breaking old habits. You need to remain patient because there aren't any quick fixes to weight loss. As with any new challenge, the initial phase of a long-term trial is difficult.

You have to realize the adaption time of the ketogenic diet plan can take anywhere from two to four weeks or more. For some, it can take as much as six to eight weeks. It takes time because you cannot instantly switch over to using fat as a fuel source. It takes time for your body to adjust to the changes. You may be experiencing low energy, withdrawal type symptoms, fatigue or headaches, but they will pass.

Make use of your slow cooker or crockpot, Instant Pot, food processor, and an immersion blender to prepare delicious meals using your ketogenic meal plan. Some recipes might not be 100 % keto-friendly. You can also adjust the ingredients to your own discretion. Remember this Formula: Total Carbs minus (-) Fiber = Net Carbs. This is the logic used for each of the recipes included in this cookbook and guidelines.

Finally, if you found this book useful in any way, a review on Amazon is always appreciated!

INDEX FOR THE RECIPES

KETO BRUNCH & BREAKFAST RECIPES

KETO LUNCH FAVORITES: SALAD & WRAP FAVORITES

Other Choices

KETO DINNER SPECIALTIES: BEEF OPTIONS

Poultry Options

Pork & Lamb Options

- Stuffed Pork Chops

Fish Options

- Beetroot-Cured Salmon with Dill Oil
- Lemon Garlic Shrimp Pasta

SNACK RECIPES

- Blueberry Frozen Fat Bombs
- Chicken-Pecan Salad & Cucumber Bites – No-Cook
- Chocolate Dipped Candied Bacon
- Macaroons
- Peanut Butter & Coconut Balls
- Spicy Deviled Eggs

Smoothies for Snacks

- Blueberry & Kefir Smoothie
- Chocolate Smoothie
- Cinnamon Roll Smoothie
- Vanilla Fat-Burning Smoothie

KETO DESSERT CHOICES

- Chocolate Lava Cake
- Cinnamon Apple Muffins
- Coconut Cream Brownies
- Creamy Lime Pie
- Lemon Custard Tarts

Beverages

INTERMITTENT FASTING

Burn Fat, Lose Weight, Feel Healthy
Keto Diet Recipes Included

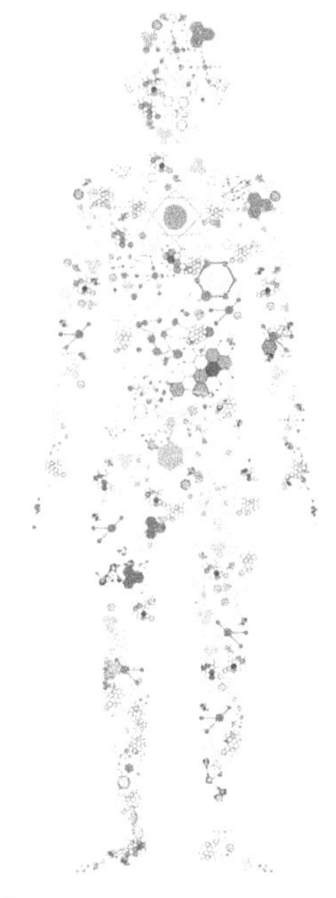

Kierra Lewis

INTRODUCTION

Congratulations on purchasing your personal copy of *Intermittent Fasting,* and thank you for doing so. I have provided you with many ways to drop the pounds using the intermittent fasting techniques and your ketogenic diet recipes. First, let's see what the plan involves for your future.

Intermittent Fasting is not so much a diet as it is a way of life. It allows you to eat what you want when you want – within the Ketogenic diet plan. However, use caution when eating what you want when you want because it can have harmful effects on your health. The idea behind fasting is to clear the body of toxins and harmful elements, which is slowing you down and causing you to carry excessive weight.

So, when we say you can eat what you want when you want, you still have to make healthy balanced choices. On your fasting plan, you should only eat when you are hungry and at a predetermined time, but even then, ask yourself if you are *really* hungry or is it something else such as boredom.

It's been observed that in short periods of time, fasting can speed up the healing process and permit the body to recover from serious diseases. Some conditions and diseases such as arthritis and lupus, persistent skin conditions like psoriasis and eczema, as well as Crohn's disease and ulcerative colitis have been gotten rid of and/or cleared up. In addition, conditions such as angina and high blood pressure are quickly eliminated. In most situations, these cases were long-lasting if not permanent.

Fasting has been around for thousands of years. It has its roots in various religions. What purpose did fasting serve under those circumstances? How is fasting done with modern-day religions? Can fasting be done for non-religious reasons?

Why has fasting become such a trend in recent years? What is it about fasting that is causing so many people to see substantial weight loss and improved overall health?

There is so much information out there about fasting and intermittent fasting that people can get lost in the information and possibly end up hurting themselves if they are not diligent and careful.

Other things to think about as we begin learning more about fasting are some of the myths and misinformation that is out there. Let's begin!

INTERMITTENT FASTING BASICS INTRODUCTION

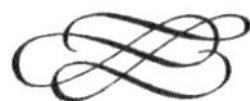

Types of Intermittent Fasting

If you are interested in trying out the benefits of intermittent fasting for yourself, but you have an irregular schedule or are not sure if it is for you, then skipping a meal or two now and then maybe the type of intermittent fasting for you. Getting into a fasting routine is vital to see the maximum results for your effort, but that doesn't occasionally mean that fasting doesn't come with some benefits as well.

What's more, once you have tried skipping a meal now and then, you can see for yourself just how easy it is, which in turn can lead to more positive changes down the line. With so many intermittent fasting options available the odds are good that one fits your schedule, so give it a try. What have you got to lose (besides a few pounds)?

The 16/8 Method

When searching the internet for information on Leangains, it takes extraordinarily little effort to find Martin Berkhan. He's a model, nutritional consultant, and personal trainer. He has made the 16/8 or Leangains Diet popular.

The technique involves fasting for either 16 hours for men or 14 hours for women before allowing yourself to consume a reasonable amount of calories for the remaining 8 to 10 hours. During this period, you should only consume things that have zero calories including black coffee (a splash of cream is fine), water, diet soda, and sugar-free gum. The easiest way to attempt this schedule is to stop eating after dinner in the evening and wait 14 or 16 hours from there. This means skipping breakfast and eating again in the early afternoon.

Again, the specifics of when you fast are not nearly as important as ensuring that you fast for the same period of time as regularly as possible. If you vary your fasting period too much, it can lead to an erratic change in your hormones which among other things can make it much more difficult for your body to shed any excess weight.

If you find yourself without the time required to eat a proper meal to break your fast normally, you should at least eat something to keep your body on the correct cycle. If you are exercising as well as intermittently fasting it is important to ensure that you are eating more carbohydrates than fats while you are working out while on days you are not exercising the opposite is true. It is also important to ensure that you keep your protein intake at a steady level and stay away from processed foods whenever possible.

The benefits of this type of fasting are that it is extremely flexible so that it will work for a wide variety of schedules. Most people find it helpful to either eat two large meals during the 8 or 10-hour period feeding period or split that time into three smaller meals as that is the way most people are already programmed.

On days you are exercising as well as fasting it is important to attempt to and always break your fast with a mix of protein, veggies, and fruit. If you generally go to the gym directly after you have broken your fast, it is important to include enough carbohydrates to give your muscles the energy they need to get the most out of your workout.

If you are planning to exercise, it is generally best to start the early afternoon off right with a medium calorie meal. Then exercise within three hours before eating a larger meal soon afterward. In this larger meal, it is important to add a larger portion of complex carbohydrates, and you can even have a little dessert as long as it is in moderation. Remember, fasting is different than dieting.

On the days you do not plan on exercising, it is important to adjust your caloric intake appropriately. Start by limiting your carbohydrate intake and instead focus on eating lots of protein, dark green, leafy vegetables, and fruit in moderation. Unlike on days you are exercising the first meal you eat on rest days should be your largest in terms of caloric intake with this one meal counting for about 40 percent of your daily total.

Remember, during this meal you should be taking in more protein than anything else. For your final meal during rest days, it is important to include a protein source that will take lots of time to digest which in turn means it will keep you full for more of your fast the following morning. It also provides the body with enough stored amino acids to prevent it from breaking down muscle during the fast.

The 5:2 or Fast Diet

For women, just restrict calories for two days weekly by having 2 meals (250 calories each). Men can have 600 calories or 300 calories for 2 meals. The rule-of-thumb is based on men needing 2,400 calories and women 2,000 calories. Eat as you usually do on the remainder of the week using the ketogenic diet plan. There are not that many statistics on this diet for women, but it is considered safe. Consider consuming about 1/4 of your regular calorie intake.

Soups are an excellent choice for your fasting days. These are several other examples:

- Baked or boiled eggs
- Natural yogurt and berries
- Tea
- Black coffee
- Plenty of water
- Generous portions of veggies
- Lean meat or grilled fish
- Cauliflower rice

The Warrior Diet

The Warrior Diet takes the 16/8 program and kicks it up a notch by suggesting that you fast for roughly 20 hours out of each day followed by one meal where you get all of your calories in the four remaining hours of the day. This form of intermittent fasting follows the belief that humans are naturally nocturnal eaters.

Therefore, eating at night helps the body easily process the nutrients it needs. In this case, fasting is a bit of a misnomer as during the 20-hour period you are allowed to eat a serving of raw vegetables or fruits and maybe a serving of protein if you just can't otherwise continue.

This works because it causes the body's natural sympathetic nervous system to activate a flight or fight response which in turns increases your natural levels of alertness, and increases energy while at the same time increasing the amount of fat burned. The large meal each evening then allows the body to focus on repairing itself and improving its muscles. When following the Warrior Diet, it's important to start your evening meal with veggies, followed by protein, fat, and carbohydrates.

This form of fasting is popular for two reasons. First, the fact that a few small and reasonable snacks are allowed during the fasting process which makes this type of fasting attractive to those who are attempting the practice for the first time. Second, nearly everyone who attempts this form of fasting reports a significant amount of increased energy throughout the day, as well as an increase in the amount of fat lost per week.

On the other hand, the relatively strict nature of this diet can make it difficult for some people to follow for long periods of time. The timing of the large meal can also make it difficult for some people to follow because of the way it naturally interferes with some social engagements. Finally, some people simply don't like having to eat their food in a specific order, try it for yourself and see what works for you.

Alternate Day Diet

This form of intermittent fasting actually means you never have to go long without food if you so choose. Every other day you should eat regularly, and on the off-days, you merely consume one-fifth of the calories you usually intake on the average days.

The average daily caloric consumption is between 2,000 and 2,500 calories which means that the regular off-day varies between

400 and 500 calories. If you enjoy exercising every day, then this form of intermittent fasting may not be for you since you will have to limit your workouts on off-days severely.

When you first start this form of intermittent fasting, the easiest way to make it through the low-calorie days is by trying a variety of protein shakes. It's important to work back to natural foods on these days because they will always be healthier than the shakes.

This form of intermittent fasting is all about losing weight. Those who try it tend to average between two and three pounds lost per week. If you attempt the Alternate Day Diet, it is critical to eat regularly on your full-calorie days. Binging will not only negate any progress you have made, but it can also cause severe damage to your body if continued over time.

Crescendo Method

This is a method that is ranked as one suitable for women since you can begin fasting without irritating your hormones or shocking any part of your body using this technique. This is one of the safest programs for women which utilize a fasting window of 12-16 hours. You can enjoy your meals for 8-12 hours. Space it out for a few days such as Monday, Wednesday, and Friday. If you have failed other diets, this might be your answer. After a two-week time period, add one more day of active fasting to your schedule.

Clearing Up Intermittent Fasting Misconceptions

Misconception 1: Fasting Causes the Body to go into Starvation Mode

Starvation is not controlled; there is no discernable end to the lack of food, and it is not voluntary. When you think about the number of meals you eat over the course of a year (let's stick to the three meals a day), is it really possible for the body to go into starvation mode, if it misses just one meal during that time? That's over 1,000 meals during the year, 1, 095 to be exact. Even if the body missed those 95 meals during the year, how likely is it that the body would go into starvation mode? It just wouldn't happen.

Remember, starvation doesn't have a determined end to being without food; it doesn't know when the next meal is going to come. Fasting has a meal at the end of it, whether it's three hours or three days later.

Misconception 2: Fasting Can Lead To Overeating

This is simply not true. For instance, let's say that after a 24-hour fast, a person consumes a total of 2,834 calories, but normally would have eaten about 2,325 calories. That is an increase of only 509 calories. Now, if that same person had eaten normally over the same two-day period, they would have consumed 5,668 calories.

The difference between eating 5,668 calories over two days and only a 509-calorie increase over the same two days becomes insignificant. In fact, some have observed over time, as the fasting continues, their appetites seem to decrease.

Misconception 3: Low Blood Sugar is caused by Fasting

When your blood sugar gets low, it can lead to shaking and sweating. However, the body has tight control of blood sugar regulation. When fasting, the body breaks down something called glycogen, which is stored in the liver for a short period of time. We experience this at night when we sleep, and this helps keep your blood sugar levels normal during the night-time fasting period.

Now, if you fast for periods longer than 36 hours, this glycogen becomes depleted, and the liver can now manufacture new glucose. The liver does this through an amazing process called gluconeogenesis. As a result, the process of breaking down fat produces a by-product called glycerol.

Related to this myth is that the only energy that brain cells can use is glucose. Not true! The brain can also use ketones as an energy source. When fat is metabolized, it produces little particles called ketones. When food is not readily obtainable, we survive and function well because ketones are the main provider of the energy we need to get through that period.

Intermittent Fasting Concerns

Heartburn: If you have chosen a plan where you have larger meals, you may need to try another fasting method to remedy the issue. Once a fast cycle is completed, you also tend to want to eat faster. Eat slowly and avoid lying down right after a meal or for a minimum of 30 minutes.

Headaches: As you enter ketosis, you may experience headaches. Add some extra salt to your diet to help diminish the issue. It will go away.

Muscle Cramps: You could be experiencing low magnesium levels. Try a supplement over-the-counter and soak in some Epsom salts. Just add one cup to your bath water. Soak for about 30 minutes for the magnesium salts to absorb through your skin.

Other Risk Factors of Intermittent Fasting

- If you are taking prescription medications, you can have

issues on taking them on an empty stomach. If you have diabetes, Metformin may cause diarrhea or nausea. Iron supplements may also cause stomach discomfort. Aspirin may also cause an upset stomach or possible ulcers.

- People who are underweight (BMI≤ 18.5) are malnourished or have other known nutrient deficiencies

- Children under 18 need more nutrients to grow.

- Individuals with diabetes mellitus – type 1 or type 2

- Individuals who experience many times a drop in his/her blood sugar levels

Intermittent Fasting & Exercise

You should work out while fasting. If you're just beginning to fast, it might be advisable to hold off on your vigorous workouts for a couple of weeks and do something lighter until you are used to fasting, especially if you are used to eating before your workouts.

The benefits of working out in a fasted state are tremendous. According to Jerome H., "You become more sensitive to insulin and allow the human growth hormone to help you burn fat and build muscle."

In short, if you work out in a fasted state, the body will turn to the existing fat stores to burn for energy instead of using the food you ate before your workout for that energy. As a result, your body becomes more efficient at burning its existing fat. Your body will still rely on stored body fat to burn for energy, whether you want a 'rippled' body or just want to be slimmer and fit into your clothes better.

There is no consensus about when to work out while fasting, except considering when your first meal for the day will be. As we've mentioned, fasting is completely flexible. So, if you are eating breakfast in the morning and fasting for the rest of the day and overnight, then consider working out before breakfast.

However, if your meals are later in the day, consider working out about an hour before that meal, whether it's around noon or even later. With the 16/8, you have a window of eight hours that you can eat. The idea is to work out in a fasted state, so make sure your workout before your first meal, whatever time that might be.

If you are just getting acquainted with fasting, take it easy; get used to fasting first, for about a week or even two. Then, slowly add exercise back into your routine. Start with a brisk walk and slowly work up to running. Next, add in an interval of weight training.

Above all else, always listen to your body. If something doesn't feel right, then stop and talk to your doctor. Make sure you speak to him/her before starting any new exercise program.

. . .

Intermittent Fasting Tips for Success

Make Sure You Maintain A Calorie Deficit: While this is true for any diet, it is especially true for intermittent fasting as it can be especially easy to overeat once you do eat in such a way that it negates any benefits you might have felt.

Remember To Remain Consistent: Regardless of the type of weight loss technique that you choose to pursue, it is important to choose one and stick with it. Attempting an intermittent fast for a few days before switching to the paleo diet before trying out a low-carb approach will only cause your body to freak out and hold on to every possible calorie until it figures out what in the world is happening.

Remember, fasting regularly and consistently is the surest way to see any of its benefits. Only after your body has time to adjust to your new routine will it then be able to adapt appropriately and begin to increase the number of positive enzymes and neural pathways to maximize weight loss using this method. Consider consistency the ace-in-the-hole of proactive weight loss success.

Maintain Self-Control: Intermittent fasting only works if your body goes completely without food for at least twelve hours. Any caloric intake resets the cycle. As such, it is extremely important to ensure that you maintain control of your bodily urges if you hope to see real results from this type of approach. Remember, fasting for at least twelve hours only allows you to each normally or slightly more than an average meal, it does not give you a license to eat everything in sight. Keeping your appetite in check is a strict requirement for success.

INTERMITTENT FASTING & THE KETO DIET

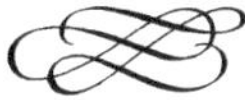

You need to make sure that you derive as much nutrition as possible from the foods you eat during your fasting. You should eat foods prepared using the ketogenic diet techniques, including satisfying meals laden with veggies, animal proteins, and berries.

Healthy Carbohydrates: You already have a very good idea of what healthy carbs are since you will be using the ketogenic diet plan, including sweet potatoes, legumes, and fruit.

Shellfish & Fish: The American Heart Association recommends you eat a minimum of two servings every week. You can enjoy 3.5 oz. for each serving by using canned light tuna or Alaskan salmon. Make a sandwich or save the carbs and have a salad.

Pork: Serve and enjoy pork tenderloin, sirloin, and loin chops which are very lean cuts of pork. Prepare 3-ounce servings to get 23 grams of protein and your B vitamins.

Skinless Chicken or Turkey: Choose the leanest cut of white meat you can find for about 25 grams of protein, B vitamins, and selenium.

90% Or Leaner Ground Beef: Get your protein, iron, zinc, and 22 grams of protein with just 3 oz. of lean beef.

Eggs: Consider eggs at just 6 grams of protein for one egg. Most of the protein is in the egg white. You can also choose a hard-boiled egg as a snack or in with a salad.

Beans & Lentils: Eat many of these as possible. Each half a cup it is only 9 grams. They are a good source of folate, fiber, and iron.

Transitioning To the Keto Diet

As you begin your intermittent fasting techniques using the ketogenic diet, you will need to distinguish between physical hunger and psychological hunger.

If you are experiencing physical hunger, you will gradually have the urge, and it can be postponed. Any type of food will satisfy your hunger, and you will be calm when you stop eating. After you suppress your physical hunger, you will be satisfied, not guilty.

Emotional hunger is a little bit different since you feel urgent or anxious and it comes on suddenly. You're craving specific foods which can include ice cream, chocolate, or any other trigger food that you enjoy. After you have finished eating, you will also feel annoyed with yourself or guilty about what you have eaten and how much you have eaten. There is 'the evidence' that you needed to hear; it is emotional hunger!

. . .

P**repare A Menu & Food Plan:** You will be surprised how many tasty items you can enjoy that are full of healthy nutrients. Be sure to properly calculate the macronutrients of each recipe you prepare for your daily meal plan.

5-Day Plan: Step-By-Step To Intermittent Fasting:

Use this as a guideline, so you have a better understanding of how to easily change over from your regular dieting habits to a much cleaner way of eating using the ketogenic plan and fasting.

Day 1: Don't Eat After Dinner:

You'll get hungry around 8 or 9 o'clock, so try one of these ways to get through the evening hours before bedtime:

- Prepare a warm cup of tea or a large glass of water versus a heavier food item.
- Use a minty toothpaste. Your mind will focus on this as a barrier to keep you from eating.
- If all else fails, just go to bed!

Day 2: Hold Off On The "Break-Fast" Meal:

. . .

For the best results of the day, postpone your meal and prepare for a 12-hour fast.

For example, if you had your last meal at 6 pm. It is okay to have breakfast at 6 am. But, don't eat until you're hungry! Eat when it is convenient. Have a calorie-free beverage such as tea, coffee, or water.

If you work outside of your home, wait until about 10 am and eat your breakfast meal after your early morning schedule is completed.

Everyone else aims for 12 noon as the time to eat, but forego the meal if you aren't hungry. Ignore the clock; you just had breakfast, so have another glass of water.

Everyone else is having a 2 pm snack. Now, it's time for your lunch since you are probably hungry.

See how simple that was! Have dinner at 6 pm. Continue the process in the previous steps and don't eat after your evening meal – until 10 am tomorrow.

Day 3: Forget Snack Time:

You just did a 15- to 16-hour fast! It is now time to celebrate!

After lunch, do not eat until dinner. These are a few tips to help avoid snacking:

If you are a habitual snacker in the afternoon, have some more non-calorie beverages. Stay busy once you leave work. Go for a walk or call a friend.

Have dinner - regular time - 7 pm. Continue and do not have anything after dinner (until 10 am.).

Day 4: Skip The Breakfast Meal:

It's really time to celebrate now. You have done another 15-hour fast, and you didn't have a snack! You had dinner at 7 pm last night and stopped eating till now without any snacks! Now, you delayed again until 10 a.m. this morning. Go ahead one more time, skip breakfast today by waiting one more hour to before you eat. This will make lunchtime your first meal of the day at 11 am.

Continue to use mindful eating and try not to eat while doing other activities.

Remember, you may just be thirsty, not hungry. Have dinner at 7 pm. Once again, do not eat after dinner, skip breakfast, don't snack in between lunch and dinner.

Day 5: Continue Moving Forward:

Today, just repeat the steps. Congrats to you! You just completed a 16-hour fast.

You had dinner at 7 pm, and you skip breakfast by eating your first meal at 11 am, did not snack, and denied it again until 7 pm.

It remains easy as that. Just select your personal preference of meal times and go with the keto diet recipes and fasting.

BREAKFAST & BRUNCH CHOICES

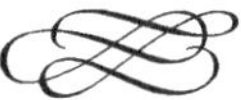

Bacon & Asparagus Muffins

Servings: 12 (3 muffins each)

Total Macro Nutrients:

- 3 g Net Carbs
- 19 g Total Protein
- 41 g Total Fats
- 460 Calories

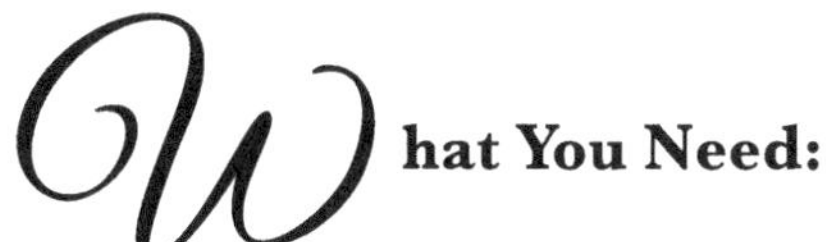

What You Need:

- Bacon slices (4 diced)
- Eggs (8 whisked)
- Asparagus spears (1 cup chopped - 7-8 spears)
- Chopped onions (2 tbsp.)
- Pepper and salt (as desired)
- Canned coconut milk (.5 cup)
- Also Needed: 12-count mini quiche cups

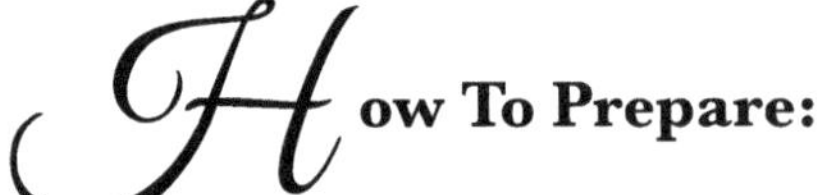

How To Prepare:

1. Heat up the oven until it reaches 350° Fahrenheit.
2. Cook the bacon in a frying pan. Drain on a towel. Dice when cooled.
3. Combine all of the fixings and pour into the baking tin.
4. Bake until the center is set or about 25 to 30 minutes.

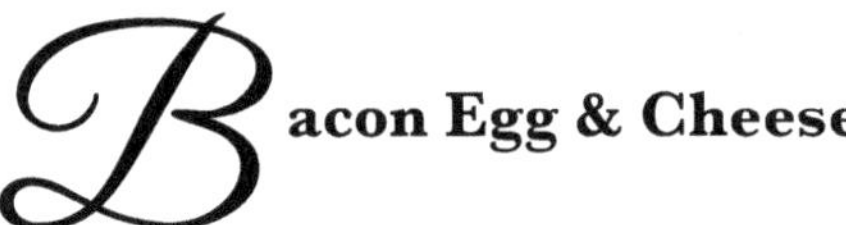

Bacon Egg & Cheese Cups

Servings: 6

Total Macro Nutrients:

- 1 g Net Carbs
- 8 g Total Protein
- 7 g Total Fats
- 101 Calories

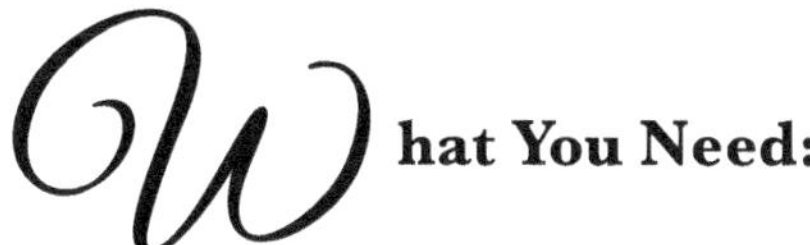

What You Need:

- Bacon (6 strips)
- Large eggs (6)
- Cheese (.25 cup)
- Fresh spinach (1 handful)
- Pepper & Salt (as desired)

How to Prepare:

1. Set the oven setting to 400° Fahrenheit.
2. Prepare the bacon using medium heat on the stovetop. Place on towels to drain.
3. Grease six muffin tins with a spritz of oil. Line each tin with a slice of bacon, pressing tightly to make a secure well for the eggs.
4. Drain and dry the spinach with a paper towel. Whisk the eggs and combine with the spinach.
5. Add the mixture to the prepared tins and sprinkle with cheese. Sprinkle with salt and pepper until it's like you like it.
6. Bake for 15 minutes. Remove when done and serve or cool to store in the fridge.

Bacon Hash

. . .

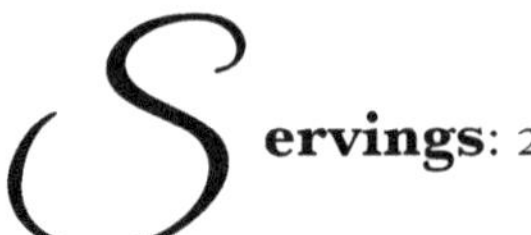**ervings**: 2

Total Macro Nutrients:

- 9 g Net Carbs
- 23 g Total Protein
- 24 g Total Fats
- 366 Calories

What You Need:

- Small green pepper (1)
- Jalapenos (2)
- Small onion (1)
- Eggs (4)
- Bacon slices (6)

How To Prepare:

1. Chop the bacon into chunks using a food processor. Set aside for now.
2. Slice the peppers and onions into thin strips and dice the jalapenos as small as possible.
3. Warm up a skillet and fry the veggies.

4. Once browned, combine the fixings and cook until crispy. Place on a serving dish with the eggs.

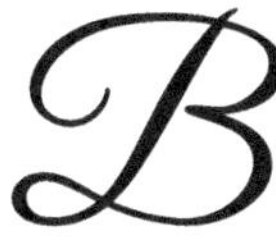

lueberry Pancake Bites

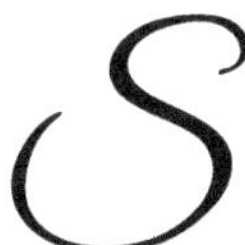

ervings: 24 bites

Total Macro Nutrients:

- 7.5 g Net Carbs
- 6 g Total Protein
- 13 g Total Fats
- 188 Calories

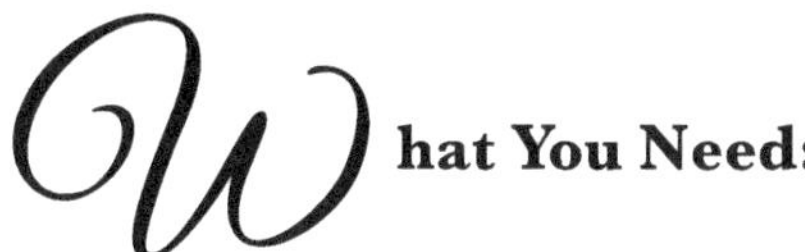

hat You Need:

- Baking powder (1 tsp.)
- Water (.33 - .5 cup)
- Melted ghee (.25 cup)
- Coconut flour (.5 cup)
- Cinnamon (.5 tsp.)
- Salt (.5 tsp.)
- Eggs (4
- Vanilla extract (.5 tsp.)
- Frozen blueberries (.5 cup)
- Also Needed: Muffin tray

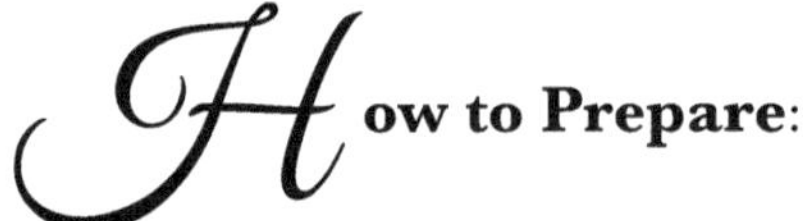

How to Prepare:

1. Warm up the oven to reach 325° Fahrenheit. Use a spritz of coconut oil spray to grease 24 muffin cups.
2. Combine the eggs, sweetener, and vanilla, mixing until smooth. Fold in the flour, melted ghee, salt, baking powder, and cinnamon. Stir in .33 cup of water to finish the batter.
3. The mixture should be thick. Next, divide the batter into the prepared cups with several berries in each one.
4. Bake until set (20-25 min.). Cool.

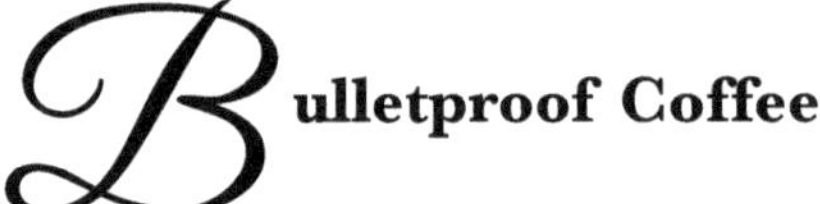

Bulletproof Coffee

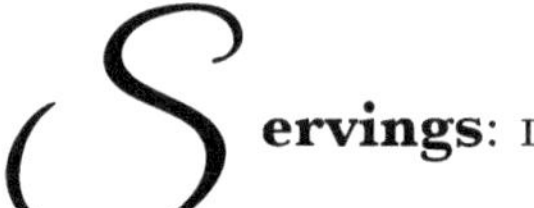

Servings: 1

Total Macro Nutrients:

- -0- g Net Carbs
- 1 g Total Protein
- 51 g Total Fats
- 463 Calories

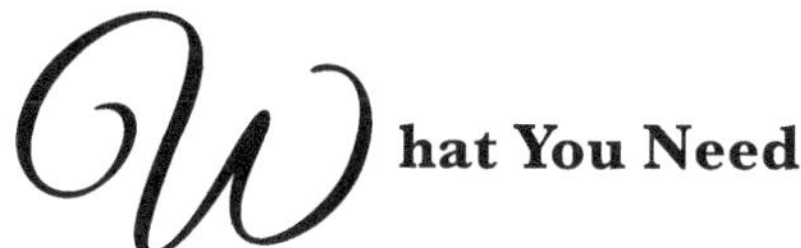

hat You Need

- MCT oil powder (2 tbsp.)
- Ghee or butter (2 tbsp.)
- Hot coffee (1.5 cups)

How To Prepare:

1. Prepare and pour the hot coffee into your blender.
2. Add in the powder and ghee/butter. Blend until frothy.
3. Serve in a large mug.

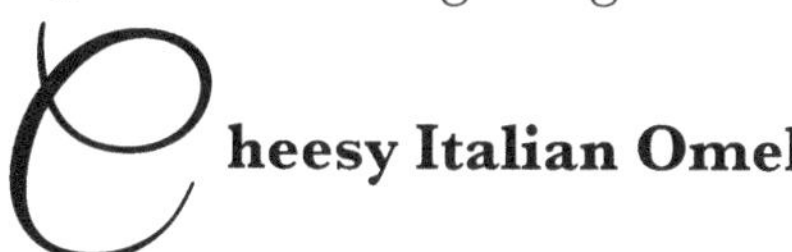

heesy Italian Omelet

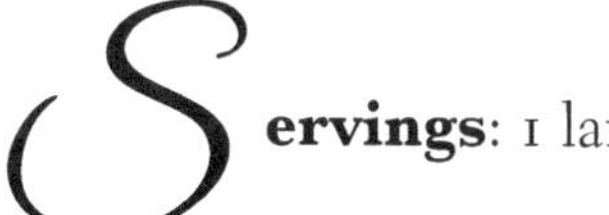

ervings: 1 large

Total Macro Nutrients:

- 3 g Net Carbs
- 33 g Total Protein
- 36 g Total Fats
- 451 Calories

What You Need:

- Eggs (2)
- Water (1 tbsp.)
- Butter or ghee (1 tbsp.)
- Thin slices salami/prosciutto (3)
- Basil leaves (6)
- Mozzarella cheese slices (2 oz.)
- Thin slices of tomato (5)
- Pepper and salt (to taste)

How To Prepare:

1. Toss the ghee or butter in a frying pan using the medium heat setting to melt.
2. Whisk the water and eggs together. Pour into the hot pan and cook for about 30 seconds.
3. Spread out the meat slices over top of the egg followed by the cheese, tomatoes, and slices of basil. Season with the salt and pepper.
4. Cook approximately two minutes or until firm. Flip and cook an additional minute before folding in half.
5. Cover the pan and simmer over low heat.
6. When the center is done, add the omelet to a plate and serve.

Cream Cheese Eggs

. . .

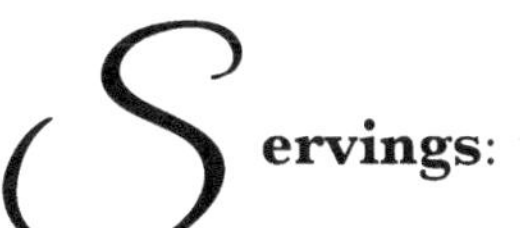

Servings: 1

Total Macro Nutrients:

- 3 g Net Carbs
- 15 g Total Protein
- 31 g Total Fats
- 341 Calories

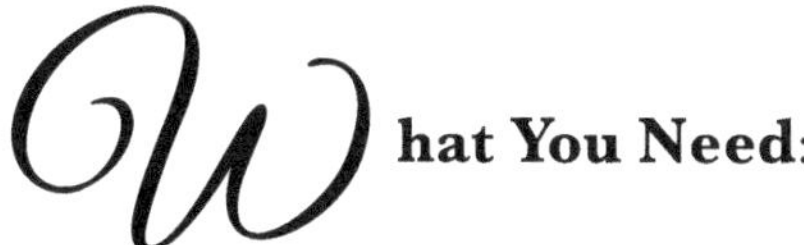

What You Need:

- Butter (1 tbsp.)
- Eggs (2)
- Soft cream cheese with chives (2 tbsp.)

How to Prepare:

1. Preheat a skillet and melt the butter.
2. Whisk the eggs with the cream cheese.
3. Add to the pan and stir until done.

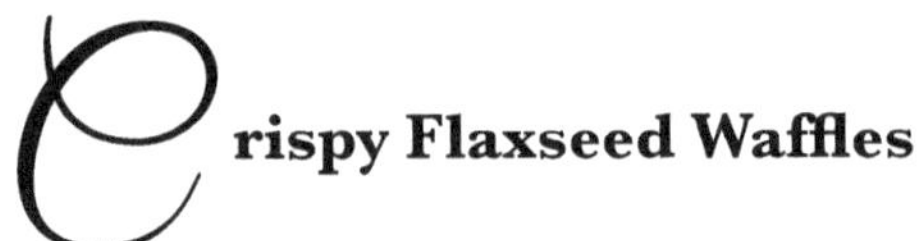

rispy Flaxseed Waffles

ervings: 4

Total Macro Nutrients:

- 3 g Net Carbs
- 18.3 g Total Protein
- 42 g Total Fats
- 550 Calories

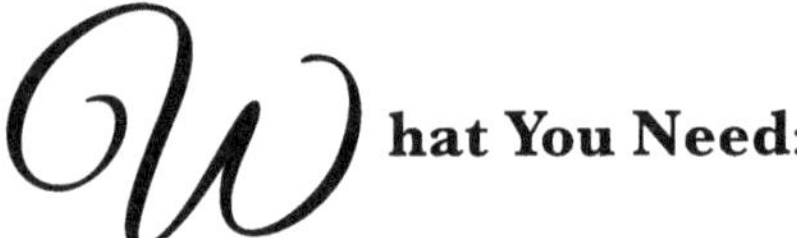

hat You Need:

- Roughly ground flaxseed (2 cups)
- Baking powder - gluten-free (1 tbsp.)
- Sea salt (1 tsp.)
- Large eggs (5)
- Water (.5 cup)
- Avocado/Coconut/Extra-virgin olive oil (.33 cup)
- Ground cinnamon (2 tsp.)

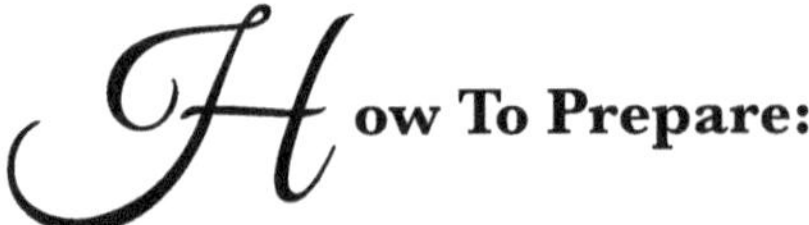

ow To Prepare:

1. Warm up the waffle maker on the countertop using the medium heat setting.
2. Combine the baking powder, sea salt, and flaxseeds in a mixing container. Whisk well and set aside.
3. In a blender, add the oil, water, and eggs. Blend for 30 seconds until foamy. Pour the mixture into the bowl with flaxseeds.
4. Stir until just incorporated and allow to rest for 3 minutes.
5. At that time, stir in the cinnamon and pour into the waffle maker.
6. Serve right away or place in the freezer for a couple of weeks.

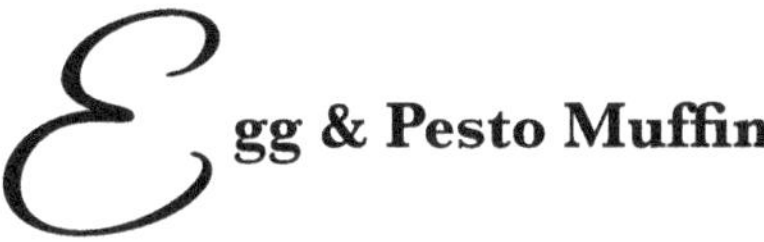

Egg & Pesto Muffins

Servings: 10

Total Macro Nutrients:

- 1.2 g Net Carbs
- 6.9 g Total Protein
- 10.2 g Total Fats
- 125 Calories

What You Need:

- Pesto (3 tbsp.)
- Frozen spinach (.66 cup)
- Pitted Kalamata olives (.5 cup)
- Chopped sun-dried tomatoes (.25 cup)
- Large eggs (6)
- Feta - soft goat cheese (4.4 oz.)
- Pepper & Himalayan salt (to your liking)

Also Needed:

- Muffin Tin
- Bowl cups

How To Prepare:

1. Set the oven temperature to 350° Fahrenheit.
2. Thaw and remove the excess liquid from the spinach (You can also blanch freshly picked spinach for one minute in boiling water. Transfer it to an ice bath to stop the cooking process.)
3. Chop the tomatoes and slice the olives.
4. Whisk in the pesto, salt, and pepper.
5. Divide the ingredients evenly into the cups - starting with the spinach, cheese, tomatoes, and olives. Blend in the pesto and egg mixture.
6. Bake 20 to 25 minutes or until browned.

7. When the muffins are done, place them on a cooling rack for a short time.
8. You can store the tasty breakfast treats in the fridge for five days or so.

Ham Muffins

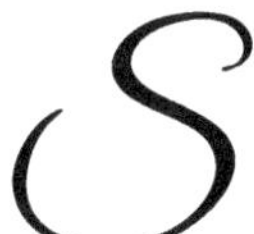

ervings: 12

Total Macro Nutrients:

- 1.5 g Net Carbs
- 10 g Total Protein
- 9 g Total Fats
- 129 Calories

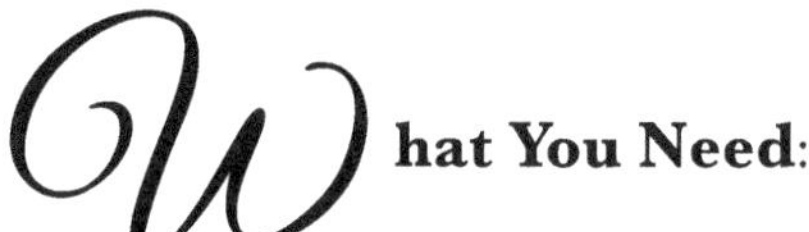

hat You Need:

- Ham (12 oz.)
- Green pepper (.25 cup)
- Celery (1 stalk)
- Pepper (1 tsp.)
- Onion powder (1 tsp.)
- Freshly chopped parsley (1 tbsp.)
- Minced chives (1 tbsp.)
- Dash of cayenne (1 dash)
- Shredded cheddar cheese (6 oz.)

- Eggs (3)

How To Prepare:

1. Line a rimmed baking sheet with foil. Spritz the muffin tins with cooking oil spray.
2. Mince the celery and green pepper. Finely mince the ham in a food processor. Combine all of the fixings.
3. Spoon into the muffin tins sitting on the baking tin.
4. Set the oven to 350° Fahrenheit. Bake for 30 to 35 minutes or until browned.

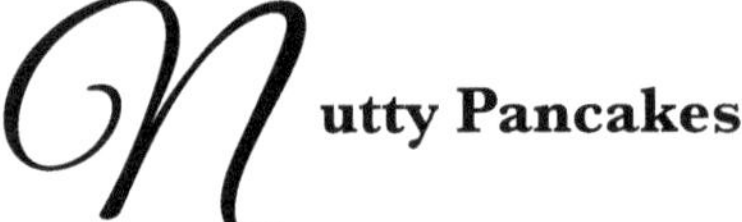

utty Pancakes

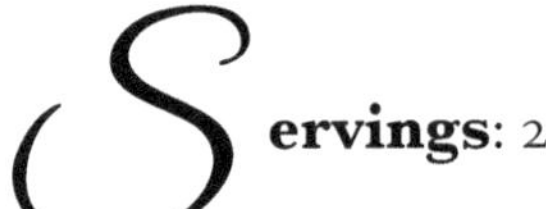

ervings: 2

Total Macro Nutrients:

- 9 g Net Carbs
- 27 g Total Protein
- 52 g Total Fats
- 625 Calories

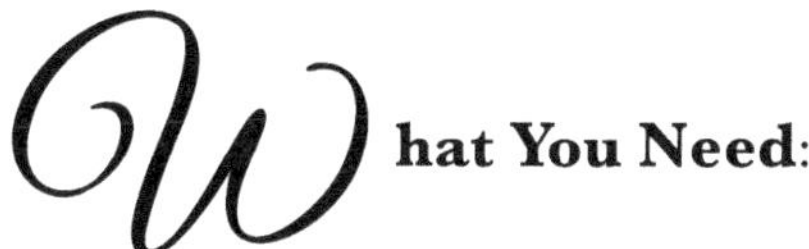

What You Need:

- Almond flour (10 tbsp.)
- Baking soda (.5 tsp.)
- Ground cinnamon (1 tsp.)
- Large eggs (3)
- Almond milk (.25 cup)
- Chopped nuts – ex. Hazelnuts (.25 cup)
- Unsweetened almond/preference nut butter (.25 cup)

How to Prepare:

1. Whisk all of the fixings in a container. Let the batter sit for 5-10 minutes for the flour will thicken.
2. Preheat a greased skillet (low-medium).
3. Measure out .25 cup portions of the batter in the frying pan.
4. Cook for 2-3 minutes per side.
5. Serve with the prepared almond butter drizzle.

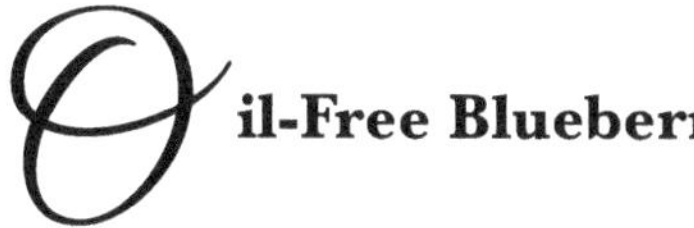

Oil-Free Blueberry Streusel Scones

. . .

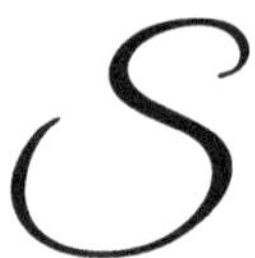

ervings: 12

Total Macro Nutrients:

- 3.3 g Net Carbs
- 0.6 g Total Protein
- 11.6 g Total Fats
- 145 Calories

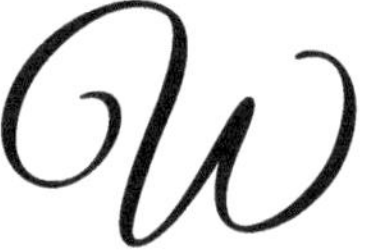

hat You Need For The Scones:

- Almond flour (2 cups)
- Baking powder (1 tsp.)
- Ground stevia leaf (.25 tsp.)
- Salt (1 pinch)
- Fresh blueberries (1 cup)
- Egg (1)
- Almond milk (2 tbsp.)

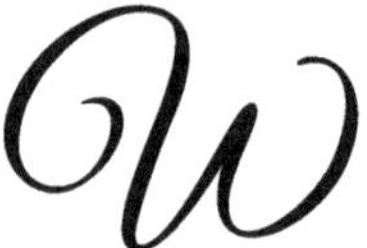

hat You Need For The Streusel Topping:

- Egg white (1 tbsp.)
- Slivered almonds (.25 cup)
- Ground cinnamon (.5 tsp.)
- Stevia (1 pinch)

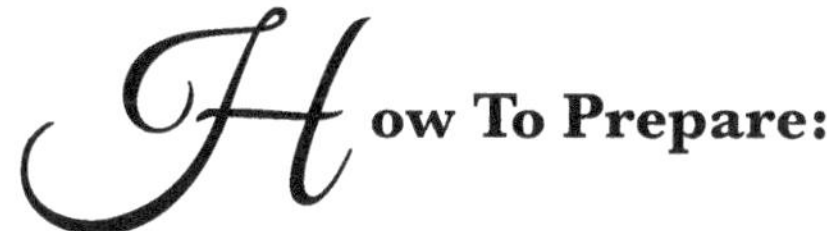

How To Prepare:

1. Warm up the oven to reach 375° Fahrenheit. Prepare a cookie sheet with parchment paper or use a silicone baking mat.
2. Combine all of the fixings for the streusel in a small mixing bowl.
3. In a large bowl, combine the flour, stevia, baking powder, and salt. Whisk well to mix.
4. Stir in the blueberries and cover with the flour mixture. Set to the side for now.
5. Whisk the egg and milk together and add with the flour mixture. Stir well. Knead the dough and shape into 12 small scones about ½-inch thick.
6. Place on the prepared pan and bake for 22 to 22 minutes.
7. Cool 10 minutes and serve.

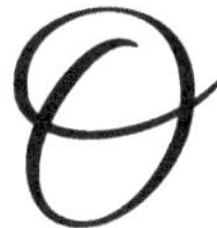

Overnight Chocolate Oats

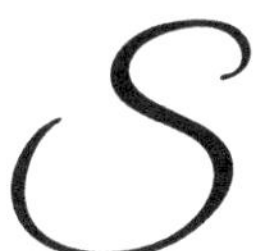

Servings: 4

Total Macro Nutrients:

- 3 g Net Carbs
- 4.9 g Total Protein
- 11.1 g Total Fats
- 139 Calories

What You Need

- Chopped walnuts (.33 cup)
- Chia seeds (.25 cup)
- MCT oil or powder (.25 cup) optional
- Cacao powder (2 tbsp.)
- Cacao nibs (2 tbsp.)
- Liquid stevia (4 drops) or Erythritol (2 tbsp.)
- Cinnamon (.5 tsp.)
- Finely ground sea salt (.25 tsp.)
- Non-dairy milk - your choice (2 cups)
- Vanilla extract (1 tsp.)

How To Prepare:

1. Add the MCT oil, chia seeds, walnuts, cacao nibs, cacao powder, ground cinnamon, sweetener of choice, and sea salt. Place in an airtight container large enough to hold at least four cups.
2. Rotate the ingredients in the container until fully coated.
3. Pour in the milk and add the vanilla extract. Stir until well-mixed.
4. Securely place a cover on the jar and refrigerate for at least 12 hours.

5. When time to eat, stir well and divide between four bowls to serve.

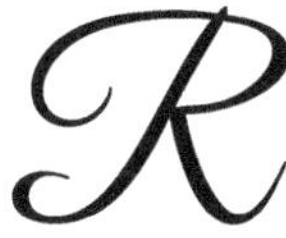

aspberry Breakfast Pudding Bowl

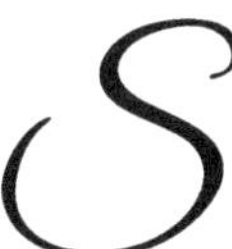

ervings: 3 (.5 cup each)

Total Macro Nutrients:

- 5.7 g Net Carbs
- 3.2 g Total Protein
- 34.2 g Total Fats
- 328 Calories

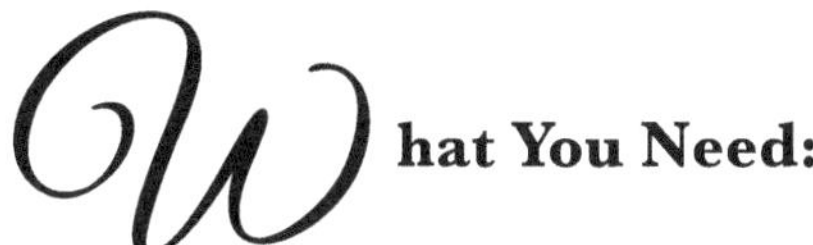

hat You Need:

- Full-fat coconut milk (1.5 cups)
- Frozen raspberries (1 cup)
- MCT oil (.25 cup)
- Chia seeds (2 tbsp.)
- Apple cider vinegar (1 tbsp.)
- Alcohol-free stevia (3 drops)
- Vanilla extract (1 tsp.)
- Optional: Collagen (1 scoop)

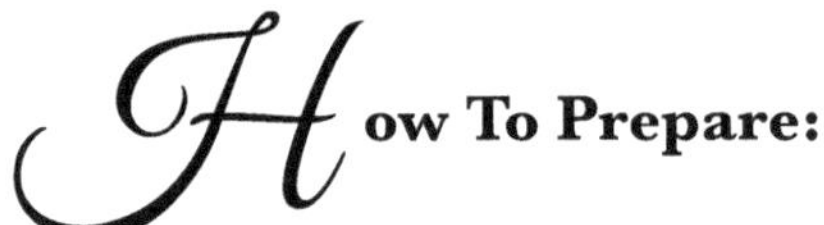

How To Prepare:

1. Combine all of the pudding fixings in the bowl of the food processor or jug of the blender.
2. Combine until creamy smooth.
3. Serve in a bowl (¾-cup size) and top with your favorites.
4. Serve with almonds, shredded coconut, fresh berries or hemp hearts. Remember to add additional carbs.

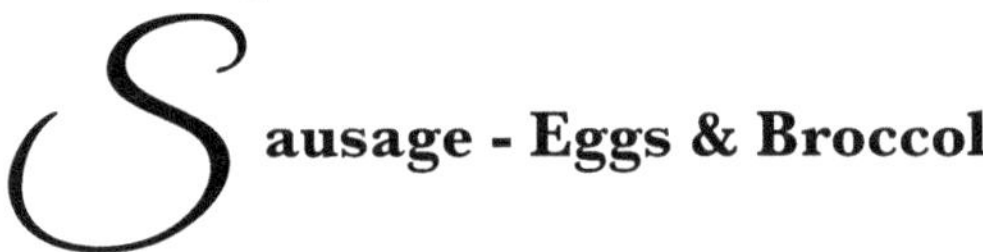

Sausage - Eggs & Broccoli with Cheese

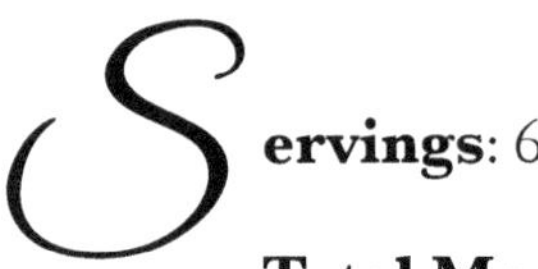

Servings: 6

Total Macro Nutrients:

- 4.21 g Net Carbs
- 26.1 g Total Protein
- 38.9 g Total Fats
- 484 Calories

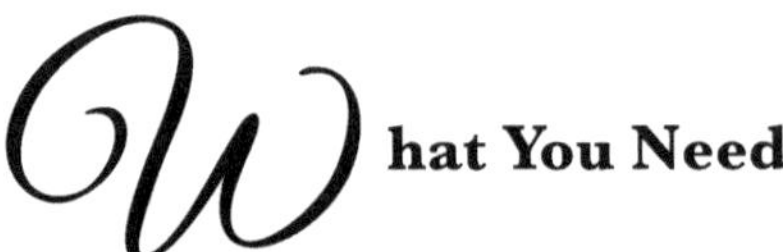

What You Need

- Medium head of broccoli (1)
- Low-carb sausage links (12. oz. pkg.)

- Shredded cheddar cheese (1 cup - divided)
- Eggs (10)
- Whipping cream (.75 cup)
- Minced garlic cloves (2)
- Pepper (.25 tsp.)
- Salt (.5 tsp.)
- Suggested Size: 6-quart slow cooker

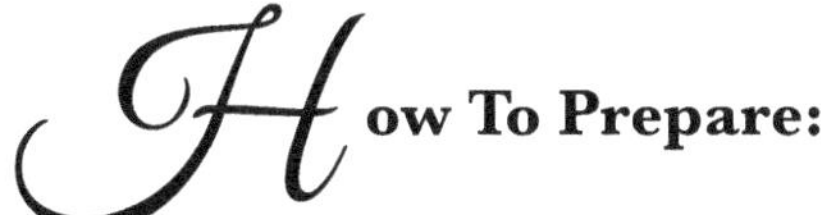

How To Prepare:

1. Chop the broccoli. Mince the garlic and slice the sausage. Grease the pot with some non-stick cooking spray.
2. Layer the broccoli, sausage, and cheese in two-layer segments (6 layers total).
3. Combine the whipping cream, whisked eggs, salt, pepper, and garlic until well mixed. Add to the layered fixings.
4. Secure the lid and cook for two to three hours on high or for four to five hours on the low setting. The edges are browned, and the center is set when it is ready to serve.
5. Note: Make your own creation but count the carbs.

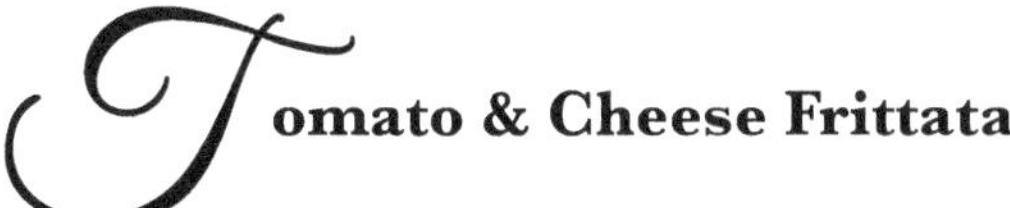

Tomato & Cheese Frittata

Servings: 2

Total Macro Nutrients:

- 6 g Net Carbs
- 27 g Total Protein
- 33 g Total Fats
- 435 Calories

What You Need:

- Eggs (6)
- Soft cheese (3.5 oz. - .66 cup)
- White onion (.5 of 1 medium)
- Halved cherry tomatoes (.66 cup)
- Chopped herbs - ex. Chives or basil (2 tbsp.)
- Ghee or butter (1 tbsp.)
- Optional Garnish: Feta

How to Prepare:

1. Warm up the oven broiler temperature to 400° Fahrenheit.
2. Arrange the onions on a greased - hot iron skillet. Cook with either the ghee or butter until lightly browned.
3. In another dish, whisk the eggs with the salt, pepper, or add some herbs of your choice. Add to the pan of onions, cooking until the edges get crispy.

4. Top with the cheese if you choose, and a few diced tomatoes. Put the pan in the broiler for five to seven minutes or until done.
5. Enjoy piping hot or let cool down.
6. Note: You can purge all of your leftover veggies into the recipe.
7. Divide into two equal portions. Serve either hot or cold.

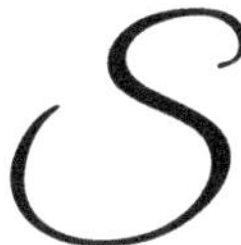

moothies

Blueberry Essence

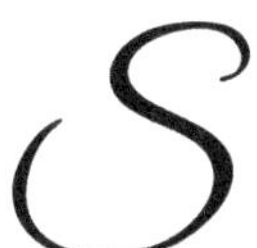

ervings: 1

Total Macro Nutrients:

- 3 g Net Carbs
- 31 g Total Protein
- 21 g Total Fats
- 343 Calories

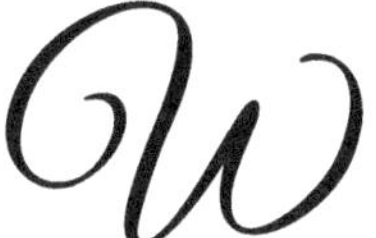

hat You Need:

- Coconut milk (1 cup)
- Blueberries (.25 cup)
- Vanilla Essence (1 tsp.)
- MCT oil (1 tsp.)
- Ice cubes (2-3)

How To Prepare:

1. For a quick burst of energy, combine each of the fixings in a blender.
2. Puree until it reaches the desired consistency.
3. Pour and serve into a chilled glass.

Mocha 5-Minute Smoothie

Servings: 3

Total Macro Nutrients:

- 4 g Net Carbs
- 3 g Total Protein
- 16 g Total Fats
- 176 Calories

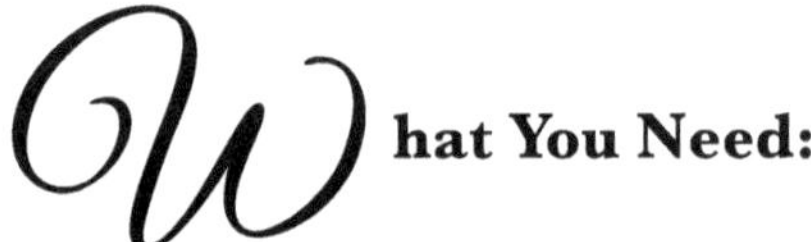

What You Need:

- Avocado (1)
- Coconut milk – from the can (.5 cup)
- Unsweetened almond milk (1.5 cups)

- Instant coffee crystals – regular or decaffeinated (2 tsp.)
- Vanilla extract (1 tsp.)
- Erythritol blend/granulated stevia (3 tbsp.)
- Unsweetened cocoa powder (3 tbsp.)

How To Prepare:

1. Slice the avocado in half. Discard the pit and remove most of the center. Add it along with the rest of the fixings into a blender.
2. Mix until it's like you like it. Serve in three chilled glasses.

LUNCHEON SPECIALTIES

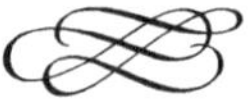

Bacon & Shrimp Risotto

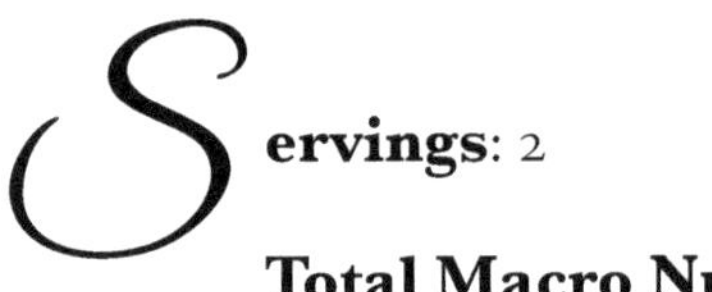

ervings: 2

Total Macro Nutrients:

- 5.3 g Net Carbs
- 23.7 g Total Protein
- 9.4 g Total Fats
- 224 Calories

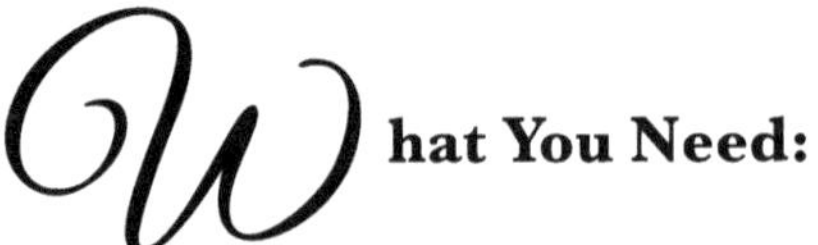

hat You Need:

- Chopped bacon (4 slices)
- Daikon - winter radish (2 cups)
- Dry white wine (2 tbsp.)
- Chicken stock (.25 cup)
- Minced garlic (1 clove)
- Ground pepper (as desired)
- Chopped parsley (2 tbsp.)
- Cooked shrimp (4 oz.)

How To Prepare:

1. Peel and slice the radish, mince the garlic, and chop the bacon. Remove as much water as possible from the daikon once it's shredded.
2. On the stovetop, heat up a saucepan using the medium heat temperature setting. Toss in the bacon and fry until it's crispy. Leave the drippings in the pan and remove the bacon with a slotted spoon to drain.
3. Add the stock, wine, daikon, salt, pepper, and garlic into the pan. Simmer for 6-8 minutes until most of the liquid is absorbed.
4. Fold in the bacon (saving a few bits for the topping), and shrimp along with the parsley. Serve.
5. *Tip*: If you cannot find the daikon, just substitute it using shredded cauliflower.

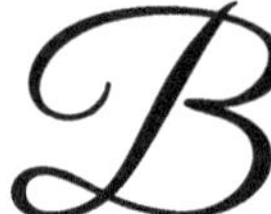acon Burger Cabbage Stir Fry

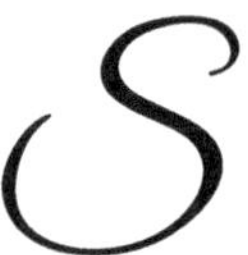**ervings**: 10

Total Macro Nutrients:

- 4.5 g Net Carbs
- 31.9 g Total Protein
- 22 g Total Fats
- 357 Calories

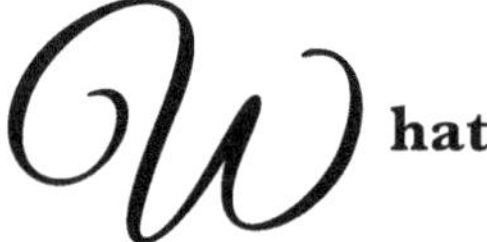hat You Need:

- Ground beef (1 lb.)
- Bacon (1 lb.)
- Small onion (1)
- Minced cloves of garlic (3)
- Cabbage (1 lb. - 1 small head)
- Black pepper (.25 tsp.)
- Sea salt (.5 tsp.)

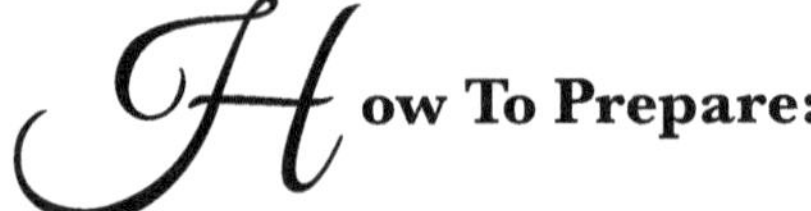

1. Dice the bacon and onion.

2. Combine the beef and bacon in a wok or large skillet. Prepare until done and store in a bowl to keep warm.
3. Mince the garlic and toss with the onion into the hot grease. Add the cabbage and stir-fry until wilted. Blend in the meat and combine. Sprinkle with the pepper and salt as desired.

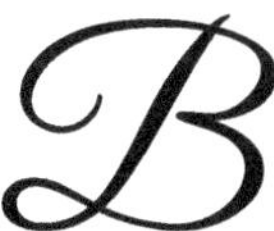

aked Zucchini Noodles with Feta

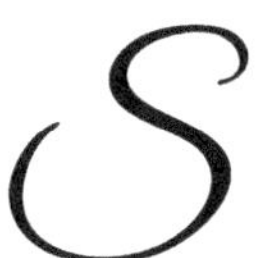

ervings: 3

Total Macro Nutrients:

- 5 g Net Carbs
- 4 g Total Protein
- 8 g Total Fats
- 105 Calories

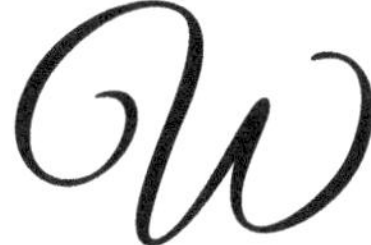

hat You Need:

- Quartered plum tomato (1)
- Spiralized zucchini (2)
- Feta cheese (8 cubes)
- Pepper and salt (1 tsp. each)
- Olive oil (1 tbsp.)

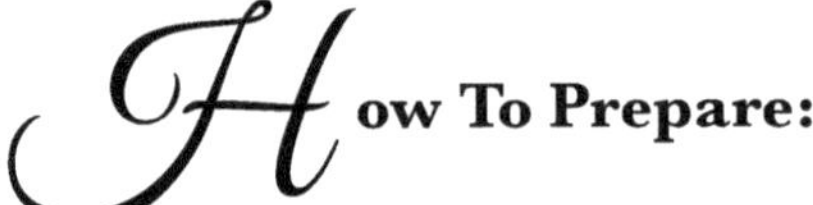

ow To Prepare:

1. Lightly grease a roasting pan with a spritz of oil.
2. Set the oven temperature to reach 375° Fahrenheit.
3. Slice the noodles with a spiralizer and add to the prepared pan along with the olive oil and tomatoes. Sprinkle with the pepper and salt.
4. Bake for 10 to 15 minutes. Transfer from the oven and add the cheese cubes, tossing to combine. Serve.

Cabbage Rolls - Slow Cooker

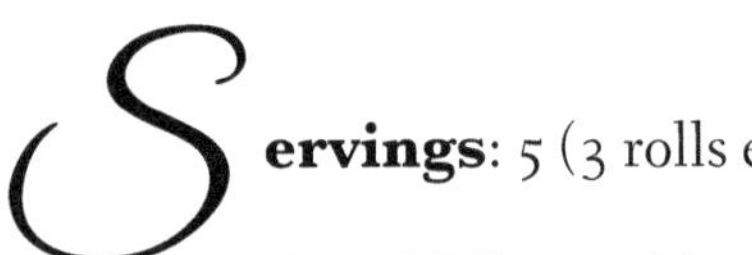

ervings: 5 (3 rolls each)

Total Macro Nutrients:

- 4.2 g Net Carbs
- 35 g Total Protein
- 25 g Total Fats
- 481 Calories

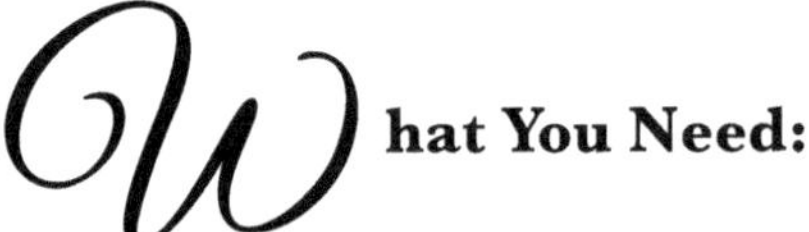

hat You Need:

- Corned beef (3.5 lb.)
- Large savoy cabbage leaves (15)
- White wine (.25 cup)

- Coffee (.25 cup)
- Large lemon (1)
- Medium sliced onion (1)
- Rendered bacon fat (1 tbsp.)
- Erythritol (1 tbsp.)
- Yellow mustard (1 tbsp.)
- Large bay leaf (1)
- Kosher salt (2 tsp.)
- Worcestershire sauce (2 tsp.)
- Cloves (.25 tsp.)
- Allspice (.25 tsp.)
- Whole peppercorns (1 tsp.)
- Mustard seeds (1 tsp.)
- Red pepper flakes (.5 tsp.)

How To Prepare:

1. Pour the liquids, corned beef, and spices into the cooker. Set the timer for six hours using the low setting.
2. Prepare a pot of boiling water. When the timer on the slow cooker buzzes, add the leaves along with the sliced onion to the water for two to three minutes. Transfer the leaves to a cold-water bath. Blanch them for three to four minutes. Continue boiling the onion.
3. Use a paper towel to dry the leaves. Add the onions and beef.
4. Roll up the cabbage leaves. Drizzle with freshly squeezed lemon juice. Serve any time.

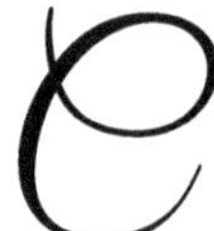

Cheesy Bacon-Wrapped Hot Dogs

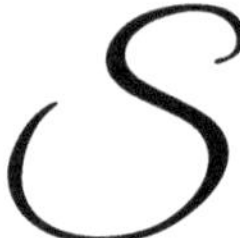

Servings: 6

Total Macro Nutrients:

- 2.1 g Net Carbs
- 13.6 g Total Protein
- 19.3 g Total Fats
- 283 Calories

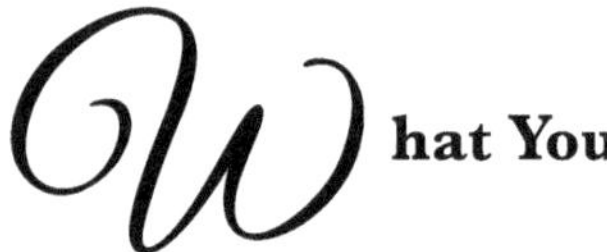

What You Need

- Bacon slices (12)
- Large beef hot dogs (6)
- Onion (.5 tsp.)
- Garlic (.5 tsp.)
- Pepper & salt (to your liking)
- Cheddar cheese (2 oz.)

How To Prepare:

1. Warm up the oven temperature to reach 400° Fahrenheit.
2. Slice each of the hot dogs (not all the way through) and insert the cheese. Wrap the hot dogs with two bacon slices each and secure with a toothpick.
3. Add the seasoning to a dish and roll the dogs through it.
4. Bake 35-40 minutes. Serve with your favorite side dishes or as a snack.
5. Note: You can adjust the time and cook them as using small chunks for variation

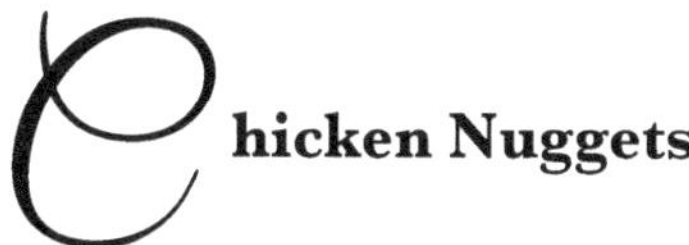

hicken Nuggets

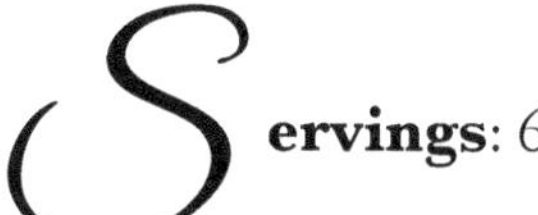

ervings: 6

Total Macro Nutrients:

- 2 g Net Carbs
- 18 g Total Protein
- 17 g Total Fats
- 243 Calories

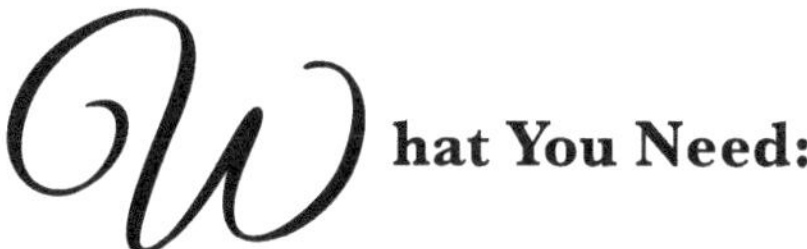

hat You Need:

- Cooked chicken (2 cups)
- Cream cheese (8 oz.)
- Egg (1)

- Garlic salt (1 tsp.)
- Almond flour (.25 cup)

How To Prepare:

1. Set the oven temperature to 350° Fahrenheit.
2. Lightly grease a baking pan with a spritz of cooking oil spray. You can also use a layer of parchment paper.
3. Shred the chicken using a food processor or by hand. (Try using a combination of dark and light meat.)
4. Combine the rest of the fixings and mix well.
5. Scoop the nugget mixture onto the prepared baking tin.
6. Bake until firm and slightly browned (12-14 min.).

Coleslaw Stuffed Wraps

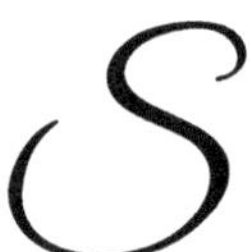

ervings: 4 - Total of 16 wraps

Total Macro Nutrients:

- 3.1 g Net Carbs
- 33 g Total Protein
- 50 g Total Fats
- 609 Calories

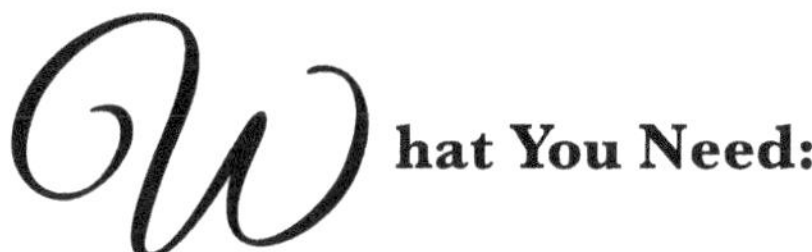

What You Need:

- Green onions (.5 cup)
- Red cabbage (3 cups)
- Keto-friendly mayonnaise (.75 cup)
- Apple cider vinegar (2 tsp.)
- Sea salt (.25 tsp.)

What You Need for the Wraps and Other Fillings:

- Ground beef/turkey/pork/chicken– cooked & chilled (1 lb.)
- Collard leaves (16)
- Packed alfalfa sprouts (.33 cup)
- Toothpicks

How To Prepare:

1. Prepare the meat of choice in a frying pan. Thinly slice the cabbage. Remove the stems from the collards and dice

the onions. Add all of the fixings in a large mixing container and stir well.

2. Add a spoonful of the coleslaw on the far edge of the first collard leaf (the side that hasn't been cut). Add the meat and the sprouts.
3. Roll and tuck the sides and insert toothpicks at an angle to hold them together. Continue until all are done. Serve.

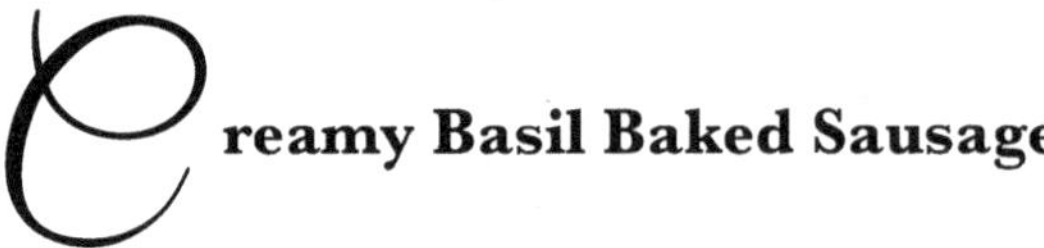

Creamy Basil Baked Sausage

Servings: 12

Total Macro Nutrients:

- 4 g Net Carbs
- 23 g Total Protein
- 23 g Total Fats
- 316 Calories

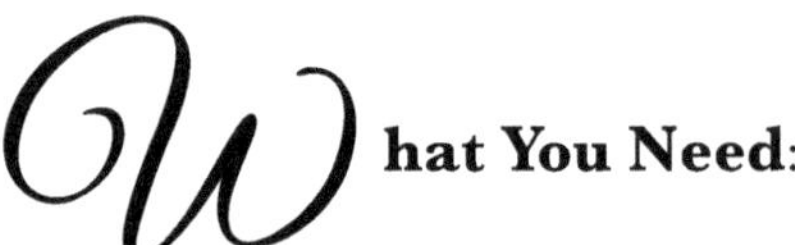

What You Need:

- Italian sausage - pork/turkey or chicken (3 lb.)
- Cream cheese (8 oz.)
- Heavy cream (.25 cup)
- Basil pesto (.25 cup)
- Mozzarella (8 oz.)

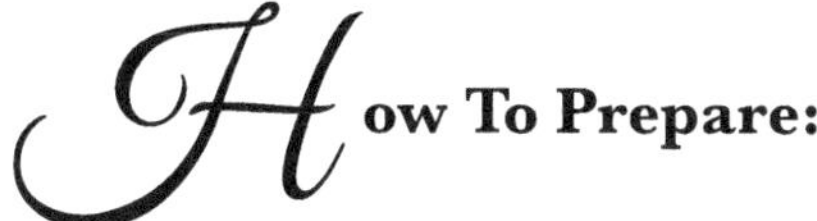

How To Prepare:

1. Warm up the oven to reach 400° Fahrenheit. Lightly spritz a casserole dish with cooking oil spray. Add the sausage to the dish and bake for 30 minutes.
2. Combine the heavy cream, pesto, and cream cheese.
3. Once the sauce is done, spread the sauce over the casserole and top it off with the cheese.
4. Bake for another 10 minutes. The sausage should reach 160° Fahrenheit in the center when checked with a meat thermometer.
5. You can also broil for 3 minutes to brown the cheesy layer.

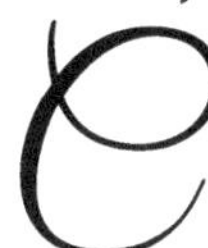

Creamy Salmon & Pasta

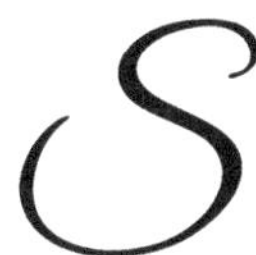

Servings: 2

Total Macro Nutrients:

- 3 g Net Carbs
- 21 g Total Protein
- 42 g Total Fats
- 470 Calories

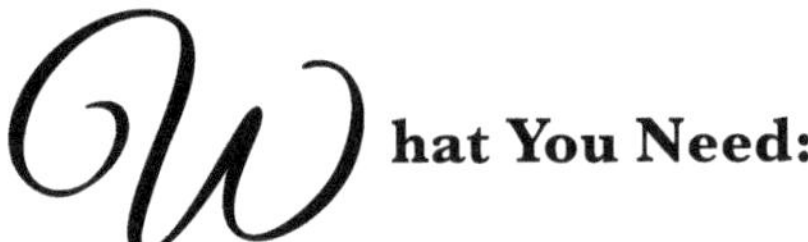

What You Need:

- Zucchini (2)
- Coconut oil (2 tbsp.)
- Smoked salmon (8 oz.)
- Keto-friendly mayonnaise (.25 cup)

How to Prepare:

1. Use a peeler or spiralizer to make noodle-like strands from the zucchini.
2. Warm up the oil over the medium-high temperature setting.
3. When hot, add the salmon and sauté 2-3 minutes until golden brown.
4. Stir in the noodles and sauté 1-2 more minutes.
5. When it's time to eat, just stir in the mayo and divide the pasta between two dishes.

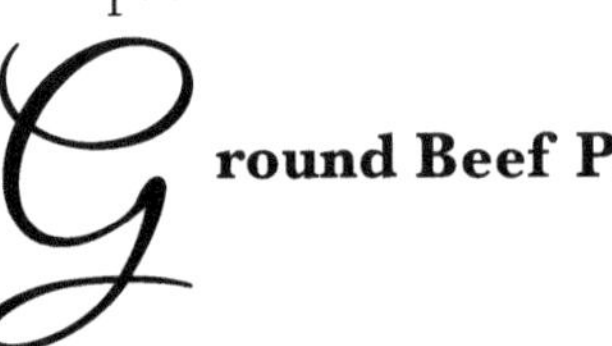

Ground Beef Pizza

. . .

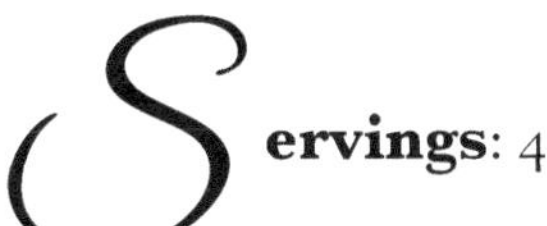

Servings: 4

Total Macro Nutrients:

- 2 g Net Carbs
- 44 g Total Protein
- 45 g Total Fats
- 610 Calories

What You Need:

- Large eggs (2)
- Ground beef (20 oz.)
- Pepperoni slices (28)
- Shredded cheddar cheese (.5 cup)
- Pizza sauce (.5 cup)
- Mozzarella cheese (4 oz.)
- Also Needed: 1 Cast iron skillet

How To Prepare:

1. Fold in the eggs, beef, and seasonings. Place in the skillet to form the crust for the pizza. Bake about 15 minutes or until the meat is done.

2. Take it out and add the sauce, cheese, and toppings.
3. Place the pizza back in the oven a few minutes until the cheese has melted.

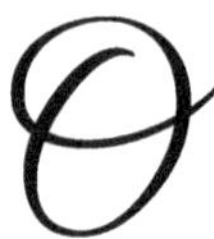 melet Wrap with Avocado & Salmon

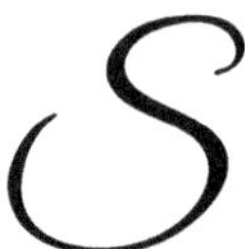 **ervings**: 2

Total Macro Nutrients:

- 5.8 g Net Carbs
- 37 g Total Protein
- 67 g Total Fats
- 765 Calories

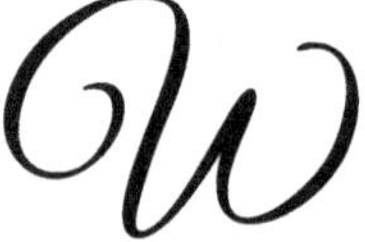 hat You Need:

- Large eggs (3)
- Smoked salmon (1.8 oz.)
- Average-sized avocado (3.5 oz. or .5 of 1)
- Spring onion (1)
- Cream cheese - full-fat (2 tbsp.)
- Freshly chopped chives (2 tbsp.)
- Butter or ghee (1 tbsp.)

How To Prepare:

1. In a mixing bowl, add a pinch of pepper and salt along with the eggs. Whisk well. Fold in the chives and cream cheese.
2. Prepare the salmon and avocado, peel and slice.
3. In a skillet, add the butter or ghee to melt. Add the egg mixture and cook until fluffy. Put the omelet on a serving dish and spoon the combination of cheese over it.
4. Sprinkle the onion, prepared avocado, and salmon into the wrap.
5. Close the prepared wrap and serve.

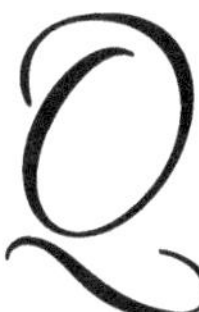

uick & Easy Taco Casserole

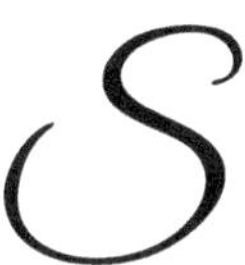

ervings: 6

Total Macro Nutrients:

- 6 g Net Carbs
- 45 g Total Protein
- 18 g Total Fats
- 367 Calories

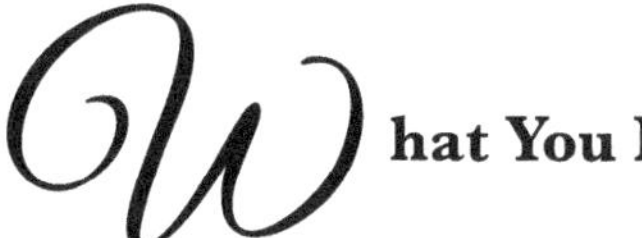

- Ground Turkey or Beef (1.5-2 lb.)
- Taco seasoning (2 tbsp.)

- Shredded cheddar cheese (8 oz.)
- Cottage cheese (16 oz.)
- Salsa (1 cup)

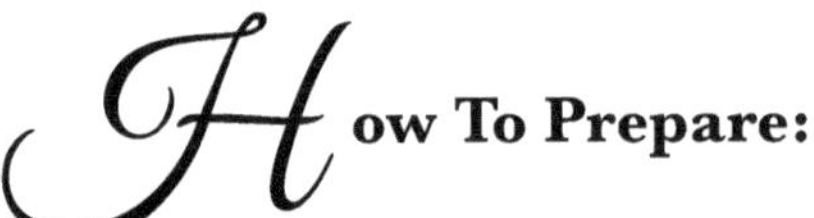

How To Prepare:

1. Warm up the oven to reach 400° Fahrenheit.
2. Combine the taco seasoning and ground meat in a casserole dish. Bake for 20 minutes.
3. Combine the salsa and both kinds of cheese. Set aside for now.
4. Carefully remove the casserole dish from the oven and drain away the cooking juices from the meat.
5. Break the meat into small pieces and mash with a potato masher or fork.
6. Sprinkle with the cheese and place in the oven for 15-20 more minutes until the top is browned.

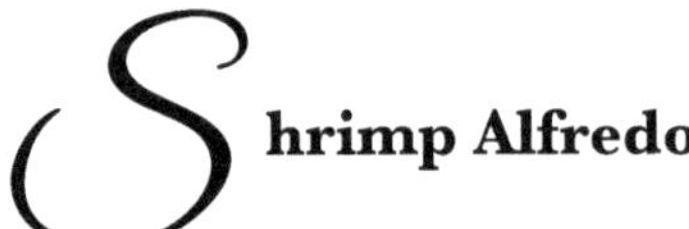

Shrimp Alfredo

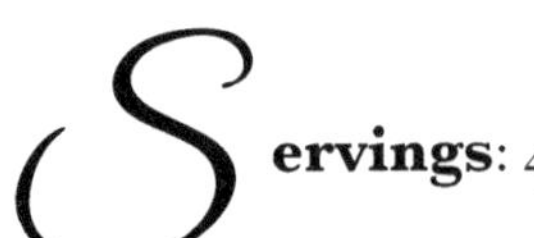

Servings: 4

Total Macro Nutrients:

- 6.5 g Net Carbs
- 22.9 g Total Protein
- 17.6 g Total Fats

- 298 Calories

What You Need:

- Raw shrimp (1 lb.)
- Salted butter (1 tbsp.)
- Cubed cream cheese (4 oz.)
- Whole milk (.5 cup)
- Salt (1 tsp.)
- Dried basil (1 tsp.)
- Garlic powder (1 tbsp.)
- Shredded parmesan cheese (.5 cup)
- Baby kale or spinach (.25 cup)
- Whole sun-dried tomatoes (5 cut in strips)

How To Prepare:

1. Heat up the butter using the medium heat setting in a skillet.
2. Toss in the shrimp and lower the heat to medium-low. After 30 seconds, flip the shrimp and cook until slightly pink. Blend in the cream cheese.
3. Increase the heat and pour in the milk. Stir frequently.

4. Sprinkle with the salt, basil, and garlic. Empty the parmesan cheese in and mix well.
5. Simmer until the sauce has thickened. Lastly, fold in the kale/spinach and dried tomatoes. Serve steaming hot.

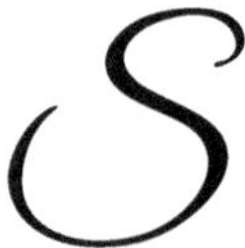

picy Mexican Lettuce Wraps

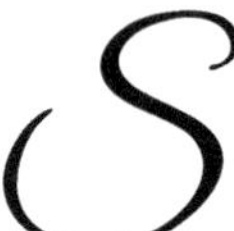

ervings: 4

Total Macro Nutrients:

- 5.4 g Net Carbs
- 15 g Total Protein
- 16 g Total Fats
- 233 Calories

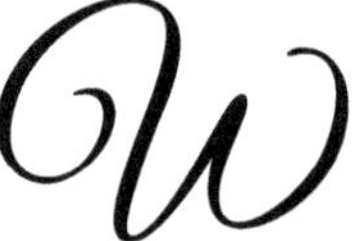

hat You Need:

- Chicken breasts (2)
- Red pepper (1)
- Hot or mild chili powder (.25 tsp. or as desired)
- Avocado (1)
- Olive oil (2 tbsp.)
- Cheddar cheese (.25 cup)
- Large lettuce leaves (4)
- Medium white onion (1)
- Keto-friendly sour cream - to garnish (1 tbsp.)

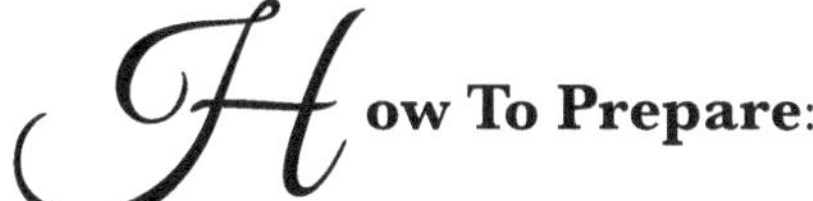

How To Prepare:

1. Dice the pepper, onion, and chicken.
2. Warm up the oil in a skillet on the stovetop. Cook the chicken using the high setting. Stir in the onion, chili powder, and pepper. Simmer 10 to 15 minutes.
3. Slice the avocado and grate the cheese. Portion the mixture into each of the leaves and add a spoon of sour cream. Sprinkle with the pepper and refrigerate until ready to eat.

Spinach & Ham Mini Quiche

Servings: 2

Total Macro Nutrients:

- 2 g Net Carbs
- 20 g Total Protein
- 13 g Total Fats
- 210 Calories

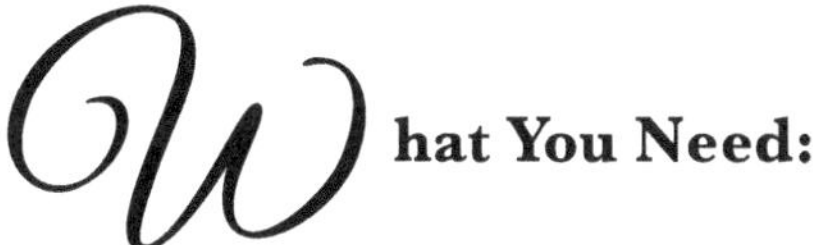

What You Need:

- Diced ham (4) slices

- Whisked eggs (3)
- Chopped spinach (.75 cup)
- Chopped leek (.25 cup)
- Coconut milk (.25 cup)
- Baking powder (.5 tsp.)
- Pepper & salt (to your liking)

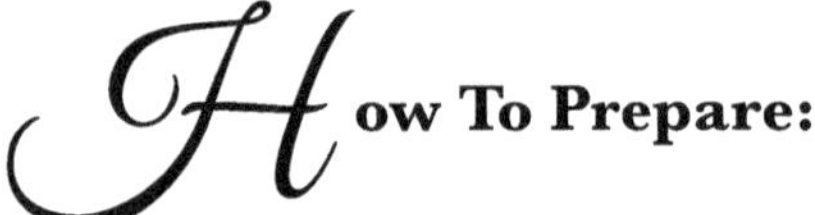

ow To Prepare:

1. Warm up the oven temperature to 350° Fahrenheit.
2. Combine all of the fixings in a large mixing container.
3. Pour the mixture into tart pans or four small mini quiche pans.
4. Bake 15 minutes. Serve.

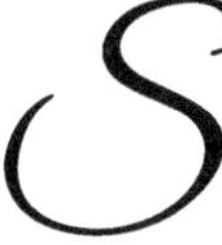

oup Choices

Asiago Tomato Soup

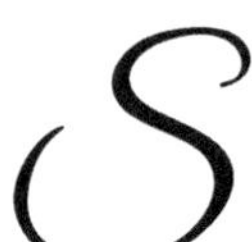

ervings: 4

Total Macro Nutrients:

- 8.75 g Net Carbs
- 9.3 g Total Protein
- 25.8 g Total Fats
- 301.5 Calories

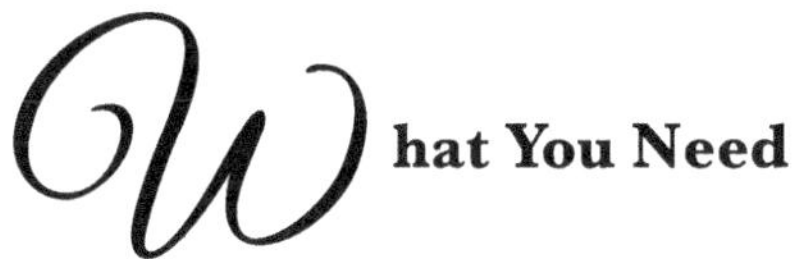

hat You Need

- Tomato paste (1 small can)
- Minced garlic (1 tsp.)
- Oregano (1 tsp.)
- Heavy whipping cream (1 cup)
- Water (.25 cup)
- Pepper and salt (as desired)
- Asiago cheese (.75 cup)

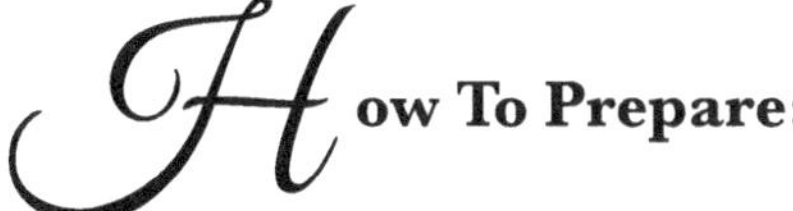

ow To Prepare:

1. Pour the minced garlic and tomato paste in a Dutch oven and add the cream. Gently whisk.
2. As it begins to boil, blend in small amounts of cheese. Pour in the water and simmer 4-5 minutes.
3. Serve with pepper as desired.

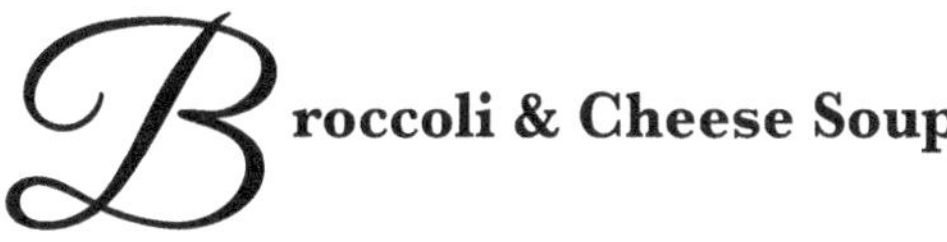

roccoli & Cheese Soup

ervings: 4

Total Macro Nutrients:

- 9.88 g Net Carbs
- 23.9 g Total Protein

- 52.3 g Total Fats
- 561 Calories

What You Need:

- Small diced onion (1)
- Chopped broccoli (4 cups)
- Vegetable stock (1.5 cups)
- Minced garlic (1 tsp.)
- Shredded sharp cheddar cheese (3 cups)
- Pepper & salt (to your liking)
- Heavy cream (.75 cup)

How To Prepare:

1. Use the medium heat setting on the stovetop to warm a skillet. Toss in the broccoli, onions, and garlic. Sauté for about five minutes.
2. Once boiling, cover, and simmer for another ten minutes.
3. Pour in the heavy cream and cook for three to five minutes.
4. Fold in the cheese and stir until creamy smooth or around one to two minutes. Give it a shake of salt and pepper. Serve.

Creamy Chicken & Garlic Soup

. . .

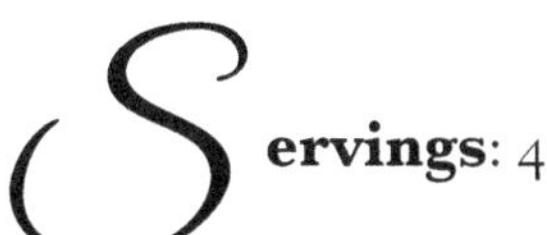

ervings: 4

Total Macro Nutrients:

- 2 g Net Carbs
- 18 g Total Protein
- 25 g Total Fats
- 307 Calories

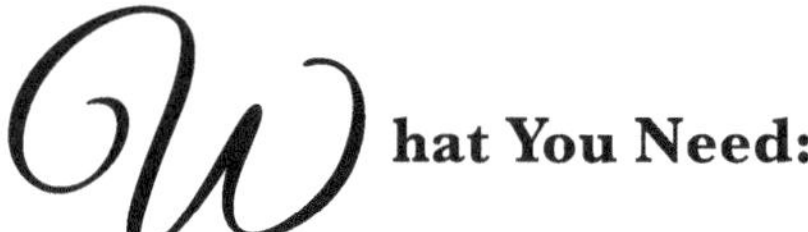

hat You Need:

- Butter (2 tbsp.)
- Chicken (1 large breast or 2 cups shredded)
- Cubed cream cheese (4 oz.)
- Garlic seasoning (2 tbsp.)
- Chicken broth (14.5 oz.)
- Salt (to your liking)
- Heavy cream (.25 cup)

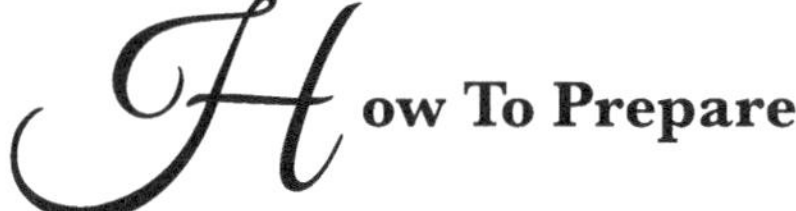

ow To Prepare

1. Heat up a saucepan and melt the butter using the medium heat setting.
2. Shred and add the chicken. Toss and fold in the cream cheese and seasoning.

3. When melted, add the heavy cream and broth.
4. Lower the heat setting once the cheese and broth start boiling. Simmer for 3-4 minutes. Season as desired.

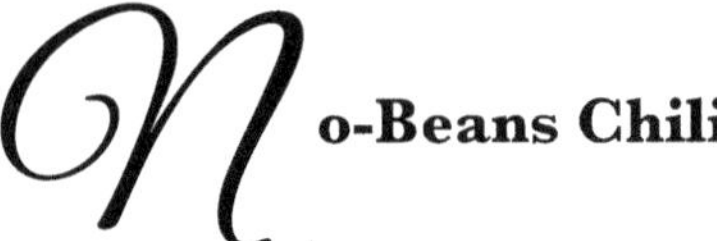

o-Beans Chili

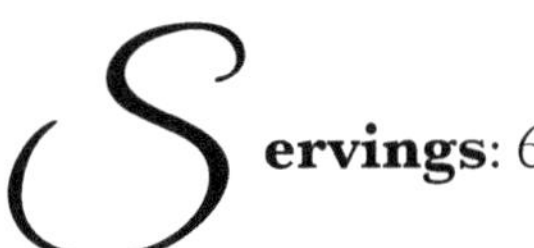

ervings: 6

Total Macro Nutrients:

- 5 g Net Carbs
- 26 g Total Protein
- 14 g Total Fats
- 263 Calories

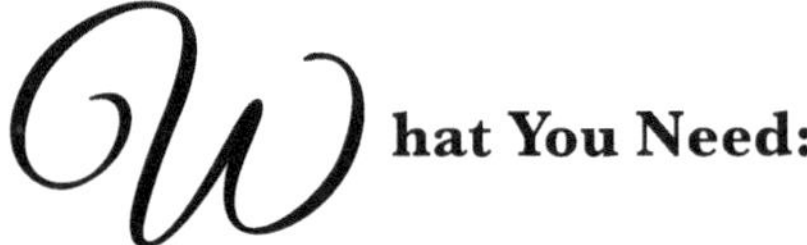

hat You Need:

- Water (3 cups)
- Ground beef 1.5 lb.)
- Cumin (.75 tsp.)
- Black pepper (.75 tsp.)
- Cinnamon (.25 tsp.)
- Minced garlic cloves (2)
- Chopped onion (.25 cup)
- Worcestershire sauce (1 tsp.)
- Bay leaves (3)
- Chili powder (2 tbsp.)

- Salt (1.5 tsp.)
- Allspice (.5 tsp.)
- Red pepper (.5 tsp.)
- Tomato paste (6 oz.)
- Sliced black olives (2.25 oz.)
- Finely chopped chili peppers (.25 cup)

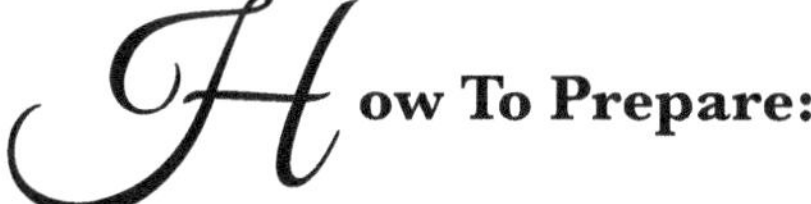

How To Prepare:

1. Break apart the ground beef in a large stew pot on the stovetop. Drain away the juices.
2. Combine with the rest of the fixings. Bring to a boil.
3. Simmer two hours and serve.

DINNER FAVORITES

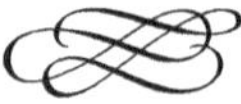

Poultry Options

Chicken with Yogurt & Mango Sauce

Servings: 4

Total Macro Nutrients:

- 3 g Net Carbs
- 54 g Total Protein
- 6 g Total Fats
- 296 Calories

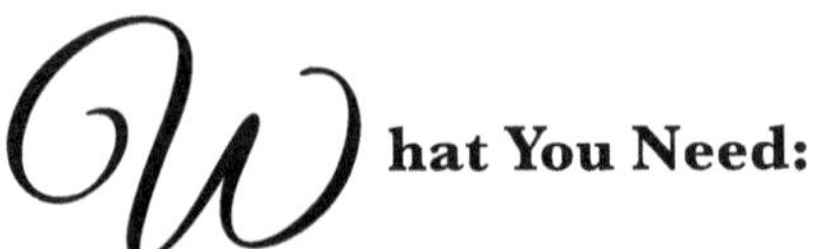

hat You Need:

- Chicken breasts (4)
- Plain yogurt (.25 cup)
- Mango (.25 cup)
- Small red onion (1)
- Ground ginger (1 tsp.)
- Freshly cracked black pepper and salt (to your liking)

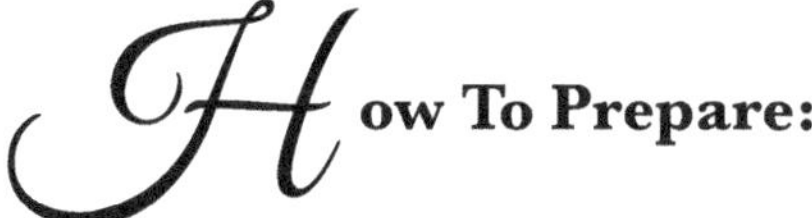

How To Prepare:

1. Warm up the oven to 350° Fahrenheit.
2. Dice the chicken, mango, and onion.
3. Fry the chicken in the oil until browned. Toss in the mango and onion. Cook for another three minutes.
4. Stir in the yogurt. Dust with the salt and pepper.
5. Add to a baking dish and bake for 25 to 30 minutes.
6. Serve when ready.

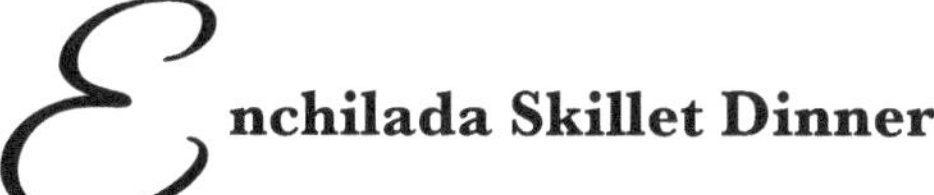

Enchilada Skillet Dinner

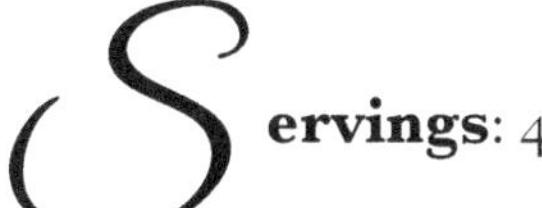

Servings: 4

Total Macro Nutrients:

- 7 g Net Carbs
- 36 g Total Protein
- 30 g Total Fats
- 455 Calories

What You Need:

- Small yellow onion (1)
- Ground beef (1.5 lb.)
- Red enchilada sauce (.66 cup)
- Chopped green onions (8)
- Diced Roma tomatoes (2)
- Shredded cheddar cheese (4 oz.)
- Optional: Freshly chopped cilantro (to taste)

How To Prepare:

1. Use a wok or skillet to sauté the yellow onion and meat. Drain the juices and add the green onions, tomato, and enchilada sauce.
2. Once it starts to boil, simmer for about 5 minutes. Sprinkle with the salt and cheese. Continue cooking until the cheese has melted.
3. Stir in the cilantro. Serve over chopped lettuce and serving of sour cream. Add the extra carbs and enjoy.

Herbal Green Beans & Chicken

. . .

Servings: 3

Total Macro Nutrients:

- 4 g Net Carbs
- 19 g Total Protein
- 11 g Total Fats
- 196 Calories

What You Need:

- Olive oil (2 tbsp.)
- Trimmed green beans (1 cup)
- Whole chicken breasts (2)
- Halved cherry tomatoes (8)
- Italian seasoning (1 tbsp.)
- Salt and pepper (1 tsp.)

How To Prepare:

1. Warm up a skillet using the medium heat temperature setting. Pour in the oil.
2. Sprinkle the chicken with the pepper, salt, and Italian seasoning.
3. Arrange in the skillet and cook for 10 minutes per side or

until well done.

4. Add the tomatoes and beans. Simmer another 5 to 7 minutes and serve.

Lemon Parsley Buttered Chicken

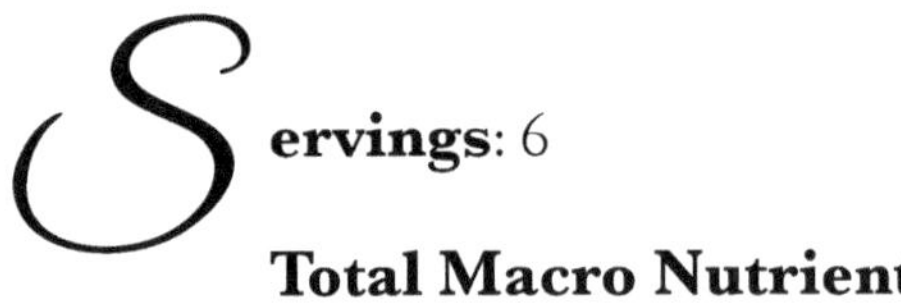

ervings: 6

Total Macro Nutrients:

- 1 g Net Carbs
- 29 g Total Protein
- 18 g Total Fats
- 300 Calories

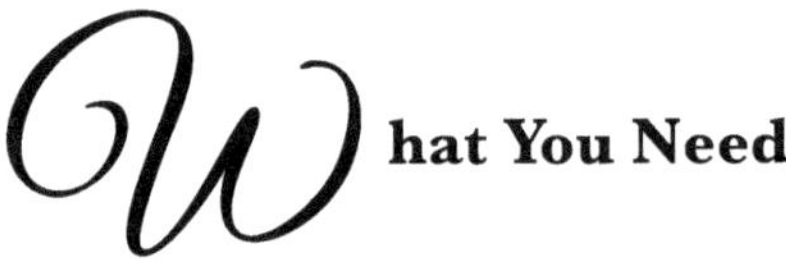

hat You Need

- Whole roasting chicken (5-6 lb.)
- Black pepper (.25 tsp.)
- Kosher salt (.5 tsp.)
- Water (1 cup)
- Thinly sliced lemon (1)
- Ghee/butter (4 tbsp.)
- Chopped fresh parsley (2 tbsp.)
- Also Needed: Slow cooker

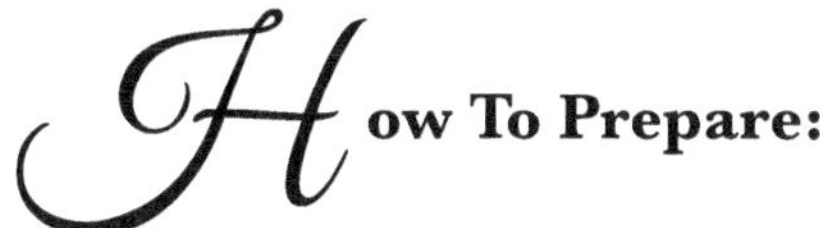

How To Prepare:

1. Remove the innards (discard) and rinse the chicken. Dry it off with some paper towels and rub it with the pepper and salt.
2. Arrange the whole chicken in the slow cooker and pour the water into the pot. Set the cooker for 3 hours or when the bird reaches an internal temperature of 165° Fahrenheit at the thickest segment of the thigh.
3. Add the lemon slices, butter, and parsley into the cooker for about ten minutes.
4. To Serve: Pour the parsley butter over the chicken and enjoy. Garnish with other toppings of your choosing.

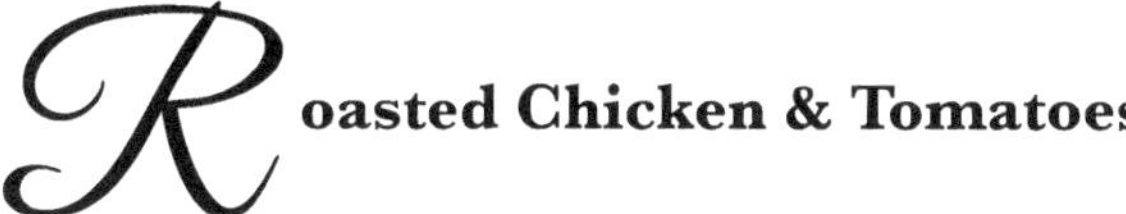

Roasted Chicken & Tomatoes

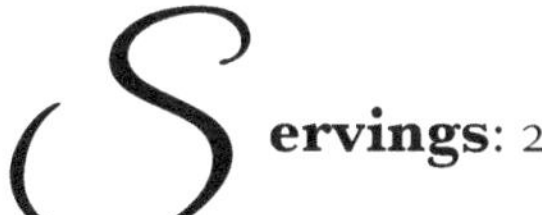

Servings: 2

Total Macro Nutrients:

- 5 g Net Carbs
- 16 g Total Protein
- 16 g Total Fats
- 233 Calories

What You Need

- Plum tomatoes (2 quartered)
- Chicken legs – bone-in with skin (2)
- Paprika (1 tsp.)
- Ground oregano (1 tsp.)
- Balsamic vinegar (1 tbsp.)
- Olive oil (1 tbsp.)

How To Prepare:

1. Set the oven temperature setting to 350° Fahrenheit. Grease a roasting pan with a spritz of oil.
2. Rinse and lightly dab the chicken legs dry with a paper towel. Prepare using the oil and vinegar over the skin. Season with the paprika and oregano.
3. Arrange the legs in the pan along with the tomatoes around the edges.
4. Cover with a layer of foil and bake one hour. Baste to prevent the chicken from drying out.
5. Discard the foil and increase the temperature to 425° Fahrenheit. Bake 15 to 30 minutes more until browned and the juices run clear.
6. Serve with a side salad.

Smothered Chicken in Creamy Onion Sauce

• • •

Servings: 4

Total Macro Nutrients (No Veggies):

- 3.3 g Net Carbs
- 38.4 g Total Protein
- 26 g Total Fats
- 400 Calories

What You Need

- Whole green spring onion (1)
- Butter (2 tbsp. or 1-oz.)
- Chicken breast halves (4)
- Sour cream (8 oz.)
- Sea salt (.5 tsp.)

How To Prepare:

1. Remove all skin and bones from the chicken breasts.
2. Warm up a skillet using the med-high setting to melt the butter.
3. Reduce the setting to med-low and arrange the chicken

in the skillet with the butter. Place a lid on the pan and cook about ten minutes.

4. Chop the onion using the white and green sections. Flip the chicken breasts. Cover and simmer another eight or nine minutes or until done.
5. Combine the onion and cook an additional one or two minutes.
6. Take it off the burner. Blend in the sour cream and salt.
7. Wait for about five minutes. Mix well with your favorite veggies and serve.

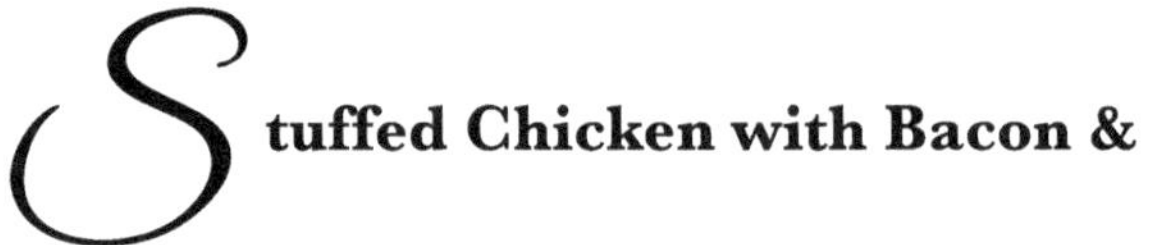

Stuffed Chicken with Bacon & Asparagus

Servings: 4

Total Macro Nutrients:

- 2 g Net Carbs
- 32 g Total Protein
- 25 g Total Fats
- 377 Calories

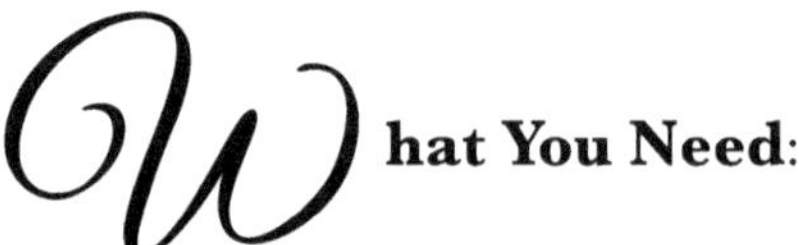

What You Need:

- Bacon pieces (.5 lb. or 8 slices)
- Chicken tenders (8 or about 1 lb.)
- Salt (.5 tsp.)

- Black pepper (.25 tsp.)
- Asparagus spears (12 or about .5 lb.)

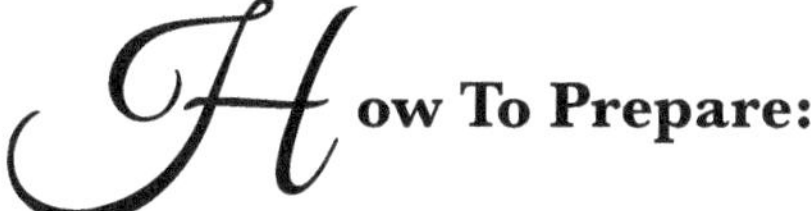

ow To Prepare:

1. Warm up the oven to reach 400° Fahrenheit.
2. Prepare a baking sheet and lay out two slices of bacon. Place the chicken tenders on top of that and sprinkle with a dusting of salt and pepper.
3. Add three spears of the asparagus and wrap with the bacon and chicken to hold it all together. Continue the process and bake for 40 minutes. The bacon should be crispy and the asparagus tender.

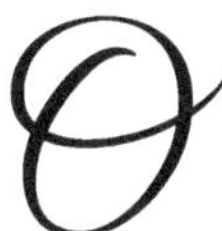

ther Choices

Bacon Cheeseburger

ervings: 12

Total Macro Nutrients:

- 0.8 g Net Carbs
- 27 g Total Protein
- 41 g Total Fats
- 489 Calories

What You Need

- Low-sodium bacon (16 oz. pkg.)
- Ground beef (3 lb.)
- Eggs (2)
- Medium chopped onion (.5 of 1)
- Shredded cheddar cheese (8 oz.)

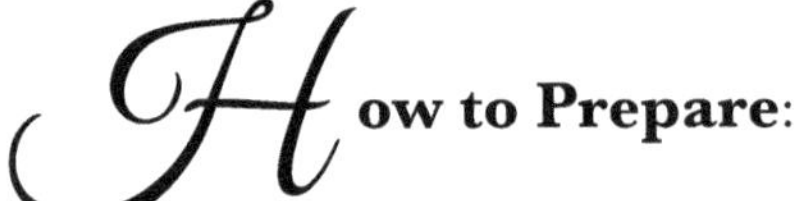

How to Prepare:

1. Fry the bacon and chop to bits. Shred the cheese and dice the onion.
2. Combine the mixture with the beef and blend in the whisked eggs.
3. Prepare 24 burgers and grill them the way you like them. You can make a double-decker since they are small. If you like a larger burger, you can just make 12 burgers as a single-decker.

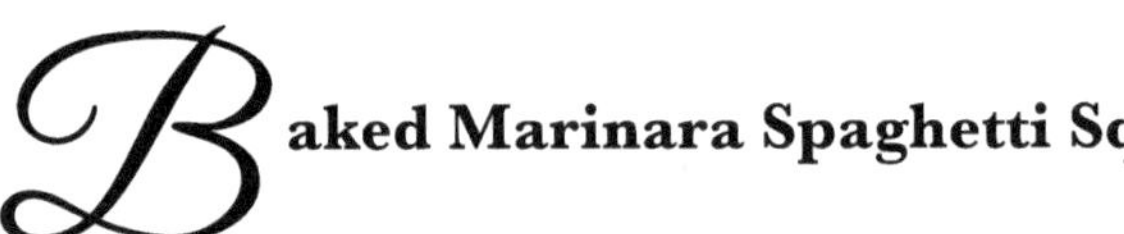

Baked Marinara Spaghetti Squash

Servings: 4

Total Macro Nutrients:

- 5 g Net Carbs

- 3 g Total Protein
- 6 g Total Fats
- 92 Calories

What You Need

- Marinara sauce – no sugar (.5 cup)
- Spaghetti squash (1)
- Sliced mushrooms (.5 cup)
- Salt and black pepper (1 tsp. each)
- Olive oil (1 tbsp.)
- Shredded mozzarella cheese (.25 cup)

How To Prepare:

1. Program the oven setting to 375 °Fahrenheit.
2. Cut the squash in half and discard the seeds.
3. Drizzle with the oil and sprinkle with the pepper and salt.
4. Flip onto the baking sheet (cut side down).
5. Bake 35 minutes until the squash is removed with a fork easily. If it's not done, cook another 10 minutes.
6. Serve.

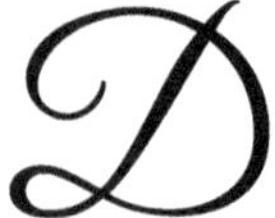elicious Short Ribs

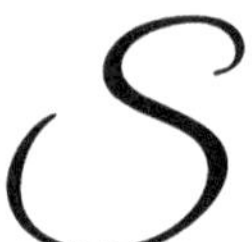**ervings**: 4

Total Macro Nutrients:

- 2.5 g Net Carbs
- 25.7 g Total Protein
- 62 g Total Fats
- 685 Calories

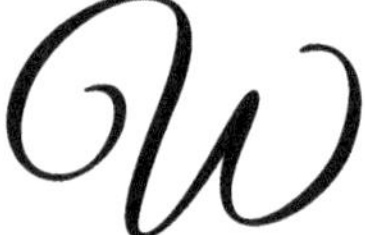hat You Need:

- Rice vinegar (2 tbsp.)
- Fish sauce (2 tbsp.)
- Keto-friendly soy sauce (.25 cup)
- Beef short ribs (6 - 4 oz. each)
- Red pepper flakes (.5 tsp.)
- Sesame seeds (.5 tsp.)
- Onion powder (.5 tsp.)
- Minced garlic (.5 tsp.)
- Ground ginger (1 tsp.)
- Salt (1 tbsp.)
- Cardamom (.25 tsp.)

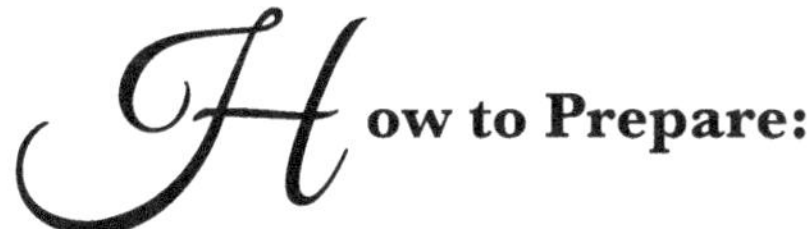

How to Prepare:

1. Mix the fish sauce, vinegar, and alternative soy sauce.
2. Arrange the ribs in a dish with high sides. Add the sauce and marinate for up to one hour.
3. Combine all of the spices together. Take the ribs from the dish and sprinkle with the rub.
4. Warm up the grill (medium-high) and cook for 3 to 5 minutes on each side. Put the ribs in a platter and serve.

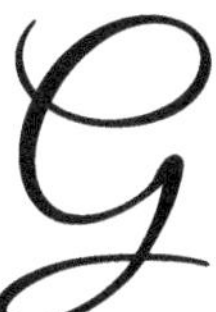

Garlic & Thyme Lamb Chops

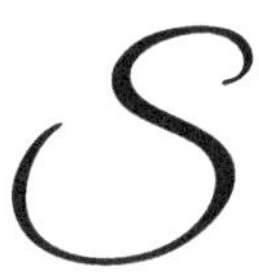

Servings: 6

Total Macro Nutrients:

- 1 g Net Carbs
- 14 g Total Protein
- 21 g Total Fats
- 252 Calories

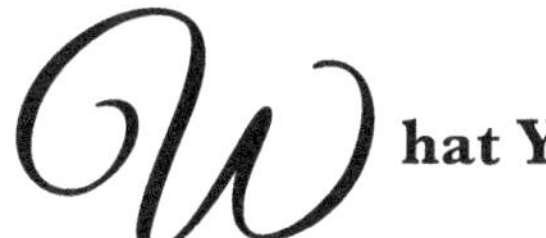

What You Need:

- Lamb chops (6 - 4 oz.)
- Whole garlic cloves (4)
- Thyme sprigs (2)
- Ground thyme (1 tsp.)
- Olive oil (3 tbsp.)
- Black Pepper and Salt (1 tsp. each)

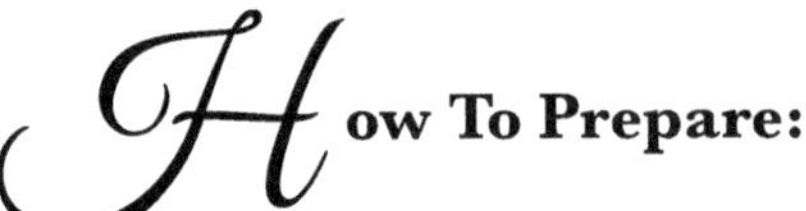

1. Warm up a skillet using the medium heat setting. Once it's hot, add the olive oil.
2. Season the chops with the spices (pepper, thyme, and salt).
3. Arrange the chops in the skillet along with the garlic and sprigs of thyme.
4. Sauté about 3-4 minutes on each side and serve.

Ginger Sesame Salmon

Total Macro Nutrients:

- 2.5 g Net Carbs
- 33 g Total Protein
- 23.5 g Total Fats
- 370 Calories

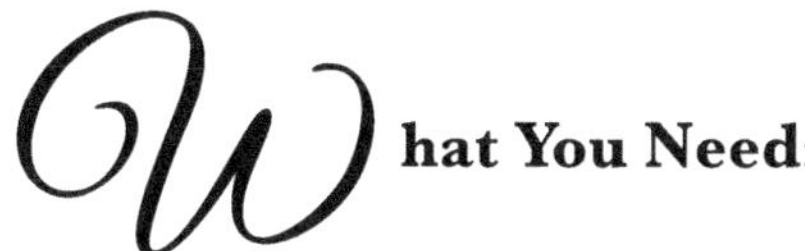

What You Need:

- Salmon fillet (10 oz.)
- Sesame oil (2 tsp.)
- White wine (2 tbsp.)
- Soy sauce (2 tbsp.)
- Minced ginger (1-2 tsp.)
- Rice vinegar (1 tbsp.)
- Sugar-free ketchup (1 tbsp.)
- Fish sauce - ex. Red Boat (1 tbsp.)

How To Prepare:

1. Combine all of the fixings in a plastic container with a tight-fitting lid, omitting the ketchup, oil, and wine for now. Marinade for about 10-15 minutes.
2. On the stovetop, prepare a skillet using the high heat temperature setting and pour in the oil. Add the fish when it's hot with the skin side facing down.
3. Brown both sides for three to four minutes. When you flip it over, pour in the marinated juices and simmer. Arrange the fish on two dinner plates.
4. Add the wine and ketchup to the pan and simmer five minutes until it's reduced. Serve with your favorite side dish.

Nacho Steak in the Skillet

ervings: 5

Total Macro Nutrients:

- 6 g Net Carbs
- 19 g Total Protein
- 31 g Total Fats
- 385 Calories

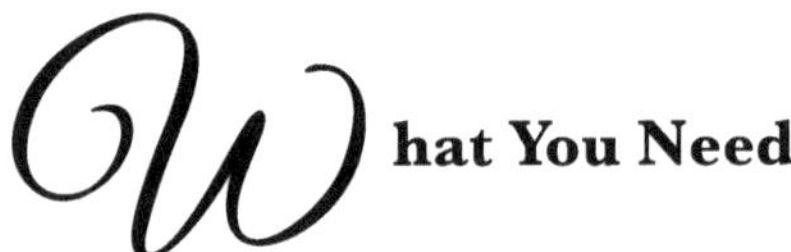

hat You Need

- Cauliflower (1.5 lb.)
- Turmeric (.5 turmeric)
- Chili powder (1 tsp.)
- Butter (1 tbsp.)
- Beef round tip steak (8 oz.)
- Melted refined coconut oil (.33 cup)
- Shredded cheddar cheese (1 oz.)
- Shredded Monterey Jack cheese (1 oz.)

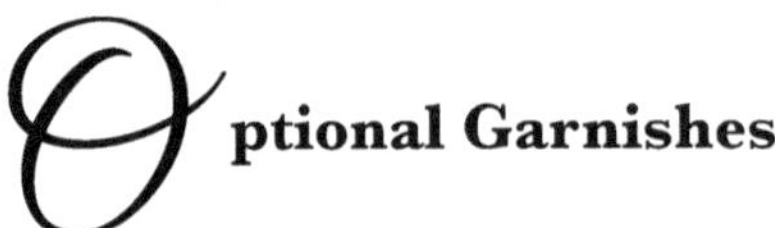

ptional Garnishes:

- Sour cream (.33 cup)
- Canned - jalapeno slices (1 oz.)

- Avocado (approx. 5 oz.)

How To Prepare:

1. Warm up the oven temperature to 400° Fahrenheit.
2. Prepare the cauliflower into chip-like shapes.
3. Combine the turmeric, chili powder, and coconut oil in a mixing dish.
4. Toss in the cauliflower and add it to a baking tin. Set the baking timer for 20 to 25 minutes.
5. Over med-high heat in a cast iron skillet, add the butter. Cook until both sides of the meat is done, flipping just once. Let it rest for 5-10 minutes. Thinly slice and sprinkle with some pepper and salt.
6. When done, transfer the florets to the skillet and add the steak strips. Top it off with the cheese and bake for 5-10 more minutes.
7. Serve with your favorite garnish.
8. Count the carbs for the added garnishes.

Pan Fried Cod

ervings: 4

Total Macro Nutrients:

- 1 g Net Carbs
- 21 g Total Protein
- 7 g Total Fats
- 160 Calories

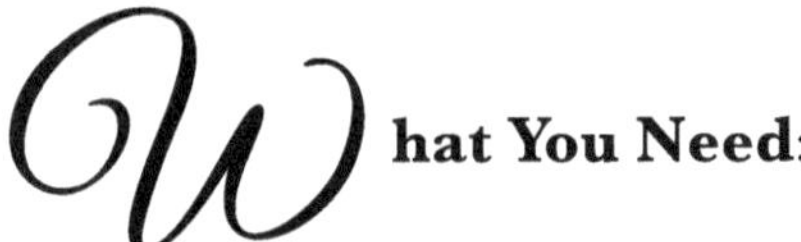

What You Need:

- Ghee (3 tbsp.)
- Cod fillets (4 @ .33 lb. ea.)
- 6 minced garlic cloves (6)

Optional to Taste:

- Garlic powder
- Salt

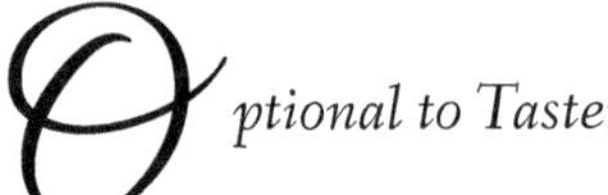

How To Prepare:

1. Melt the ghee and about half of the garlic into a skillet.
2. Arrange the fillets in the pan using the medium-high heat setting. Sprinkle with the garlic powder, pepper, and the salt.
3. Once it turns white halfway up its side, turn it over, and add the remainder of the minced garlic. Continue cooking until it flakes easily.
4. Serve with some ghee-garlic from the pan.

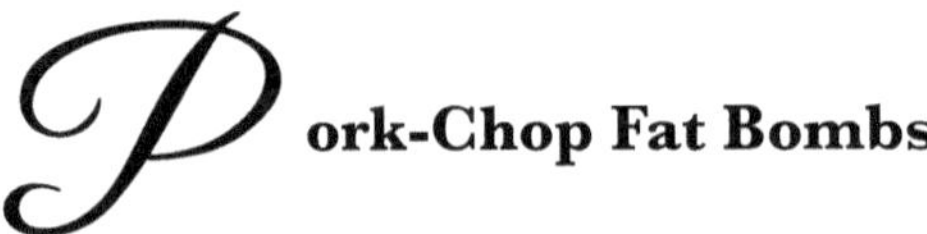

Pork-Chop Fat Bombs

. . .

ervings: 3

Total Macro Nutrients:

- 7 g Net Carbs
- 30 g Total Protein
- 103 g Total Fats
- 1076 Calories

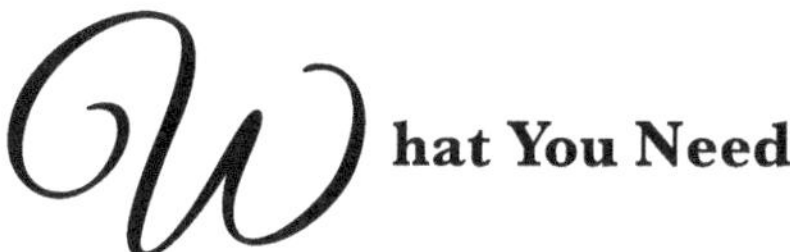

hat You Need

- Boneless pork chops (3)
- Oil (.5 cup)
- Medium yellow onion (1)
- Brown mushrooms (8 oz.)
- Nutmeg (1 tsp.)
- Garlic powder (1 tsp.)
- Balsamic vinegar (1 tbsp.)
- Mayonnaise (1 cup)

How To Prepare:

1. Rinse, drain, and slice the mushrooms. Peel and slice the

onion. Put them in a large skillet with the oil and sauté until wilted.

2. Place the chops to the side and sprinkle with the nutmeg and garlic powder. Cook until done. Transfer the prepared chops onto a plate.
3. Whisk in the vinegar and mayonnaise into the pan. The thick sauce can be thinned with a bit of chicken broth if needed. (Add 2 tablespoons at a time.)
4. Ladle the sauce over the bomb and serve.

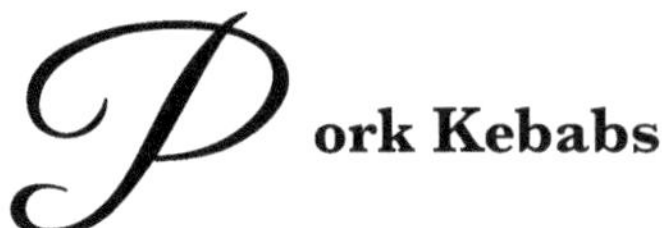

ork Kebabs

ervings: 4

Total Macro Nutrients:

- 3.3 g Net Carbs
- 33.7 g Total Protein
- 8.6 g Total Fats

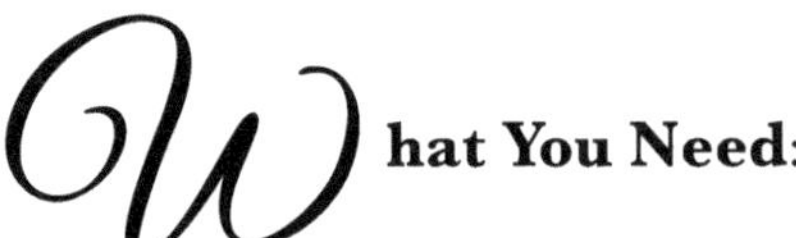

hat You Need:

- Hot sauce (2 tsp.)
- Sunflower seed butter (3 tbsp.)
- Minced garlic (1 tbsp.)
- Keto-friendly soy sauce (1 tbsp.)
- Water (1 tbsp.)

- Medium green pepper (1)
- Crushed red pepper (.5 tsp.)
- Squared pork for kebabs (1 lb.)

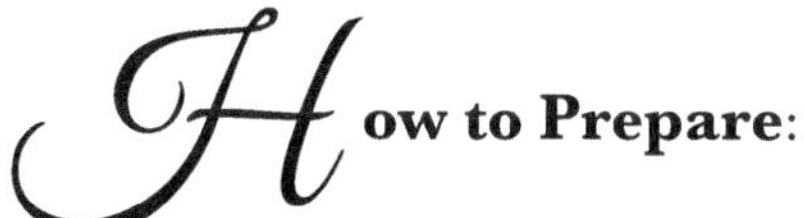

ow to Prepare:

1. Warm up the oven or grill using the broil or the high heat setting.
2. In a processor or blender, combine the water with the red pepper, soy sauce, garlic, butter, and hot sauce.
3. Slice the pork into squares. Cover with the marinade and rest for one hour.
4. Chop the peppers to fit the skewer. Thread the skewers alternating the pork and peppers.
5. Broil using the high heat setting for five minutes per side.

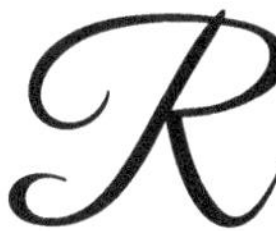

oasted Leg of Lamb

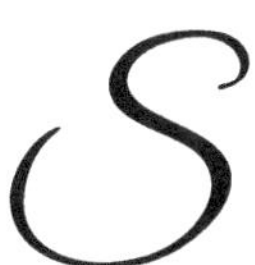

ervings: 2

Total Macro Nutrients:

- 1 g Net Carbs
- 22 g Total Protein
- 14 g Total Fats
- 223 Calories

What You Need:

- Reduced-sodium beef broth (.5 cup)
- Leg of lamb (2 lb.)
- Chopped garlic cloves (6)
- Fresh rosemary leaves (1 tbsp.)
- Black pepper (1 tsp.)
- Salt (2 tsp.)

How To Prepare:

1. Grease a baking pan and set the oven temperature to 400° Fahrenheit.
2. Arrange the lamb in the pan and add the broth and seasonings.
3. Roast 30 minutes and lower the heat to 350° Fahrenheit. Continue cooking for about one hour or until done.
4. Let the lamb stand about 20 minutes before slicing to serve.
5. Enjoy with some roasted Brussels sprouts and extra rosemary for a tasty change of pace.

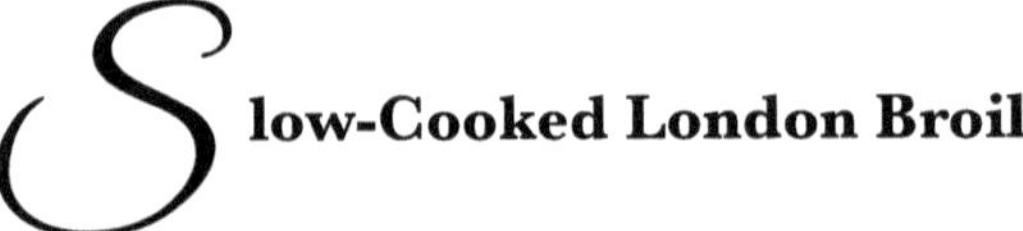

Slow-Cooked London Broil

. . .

Servings: 4

Total Macro Nutrients:

- 2.6 g Net Carbs
- 47.3 g Total Protein
- 18.3 g Total Fats
- 409 Calories

What You Need

- London broil (2 lb.)
- Dijon mustard (1 tbsp.)
- Reduced sugar ketchup (2 tbsp.)
- Coconut Aminos or your favorite soy sauce substitute (2 tbsp.)
- Coffee (.5 cup)
- Chicken broth (.5 cup)
- White wine (.25 cup)
- Onion powder (2 tsp.)
- Minced garlic (2 tsp.)

How To Prepare:

1. Arrange the beef in the cooker. Cover both sides with the mustard, soy sauce, ketchup, and minced garlic.
2. Pour the liquids into the cooker and give it a sprinkle of the onion powder.
3. Cook for four to six hours. When the timer buzzes, shred the meat. Combine with the juices and serve.

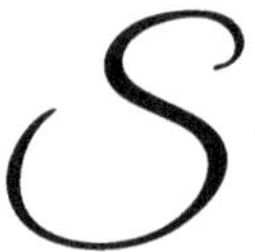

tuffed Pork Tenderloin

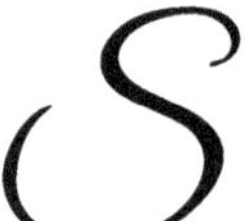

ervings: 6

Total Macro Nutrients:

- 2.9 g Net Carbs
- 28.8 g Total Protein
- 6.2 g Total Fats
- 194 Calories

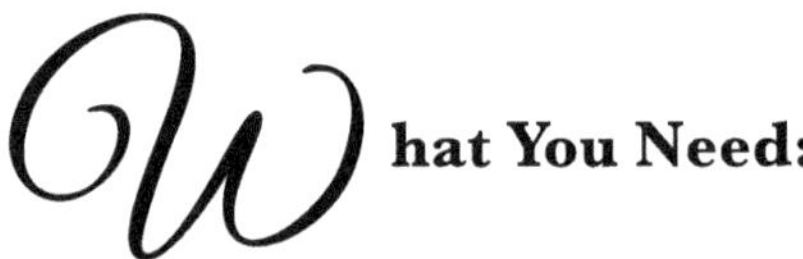

- Pork tenderloin or venison (2 lb.)
- Feta cheese (.5 cup)
- Gorgonzola cheese (.5 cup)
- Chopped onion (1 tsp.)
- Minced garlic (2 cloves)
- Crushed almonds (2 tbsp.)
- Sea Salt & black pepper (.5 tsp. each)

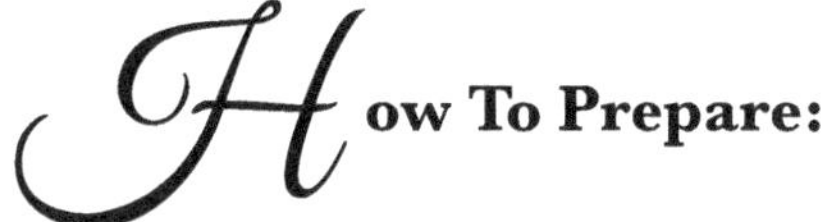

How To Prepare:

1. Warm up the grill. Create a pocket in the tenderloin using a sharp knife.
2. Combine the cheeses, onions, almonds, and garlic.
3. Stuff the pork pocket and seal using a skewer.
4. Grill until done with the lid closed (about 300-350° Fahrenheit). The center of the meat should reach 150° Fahrenheit.)
5. Let it rest about 15 minutes tented with foil before serving.

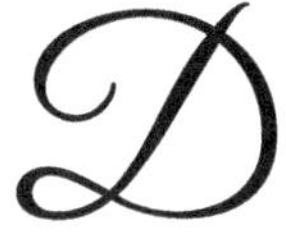

Delicious Sides

Caprese Skewers

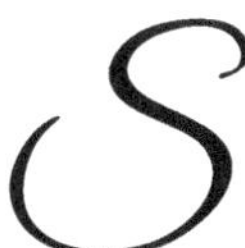

Servings: 2

Total Macro Nutrients:

- 7 g Net Carbs
- 24.5 g Total Protein
- 27.4 g Total Fats
- 384 Calories

What You Need:

- Baby mozzarella cheese balls (2 cups)
- Cherry or baby heirloom tomatoes (2 cups)
- Pitted mixed olives (.5 cup)
- Green/red pesto (2 tbsp.)
- Fresh basil (2 tbsp.)

How To Prepare:

1. Rinse the basil and tomatoes.
2. Marinate the kalamata and green olives in extra-virgin olive oil with the oregano.
3. Combine the mozzarella with the pesto.
4. Arrange the olives, mozzarella, and tomatoes onto the skewers and garnish with the basil.
5. Serve any time.

Mock Mac 'N' Cheese

ervings: 4

Total Macro Nutrients:

- 7 g Net Carbs
- 11 g Total Protein

- 23 g Total Fats
- 294 Calories

What You Need:

- Cauliflower (1 head)
- Butter (3 tbsp.)
- Unsweetened almond milk (.25 cup)
- Heavy cream (.25 cup)
- Cheddar cheese (1 cup)
- Freshly cracked black pepper & Sea salt (as desired)

How To Prepare:

1. Use a sharp knife to slice the cauliflower into small florets. Shred the cheese.
2. Prepare the oven to reach 450° Fahrenheit. Cover a baking sheet with a layer of parchment paper or foil.
3. Melt 2 tbsp. of the butter in a saucepan. Toss the florets and butter together. Sprinkle with the pepper and salt. Place the cauliflower on the baking pan and roast 10-15 minutes.
4. Warm up the rest of the butter, milk, heavy cream, and cheese in the microwave or double boiler. Pour the cheese over the cauliflower and serve.

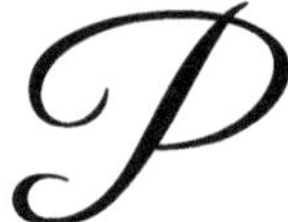

armesan Onion Rings

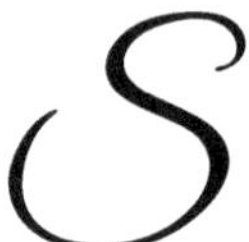

ervings: 4

Total Macro Nutrients:

- 5 g Net Carbs
- 3 g Total Protein
- 7 g Total Fats
- 89 Calories

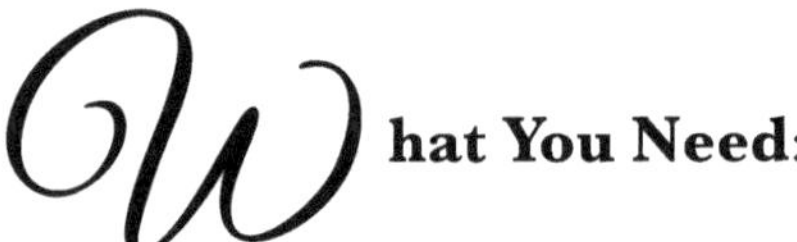

hat You Need:

- Large white onion (1)
- Medium egg (1)
- Pepper to taste
- Parmesan cheese (1 tbsp.)
- Coconut flour (1 tbsp.)
- Heavy cream (1 tbsp.)
- Olive oil – for frying

How To Prepare:

1. In a skillet, warm the oil until it reaches 350° Fahrenheit.

2. Slice the onions into thick rings.
3. Whisk the flour, cheese, and pepper.
4. Whisk the cream and egg together.
5. Dip the sliced rings into the wet and then the dry mixture. Gently add to the oil. Cook for two to three minutes. Drain on a towel-lined platter. Serve while hot.

Roasted Veggies

ervings: 6

Total Macro Nutrients:

- 3 g Net Carbs
- 2 g Total Protein
- 5 g Total Fats
- 65 Calories

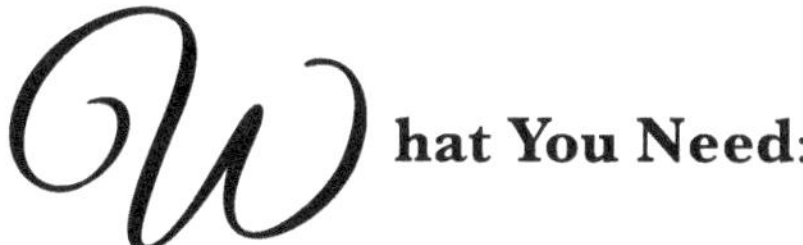

hat You Need:

- Button mushrooms (1 cup)
- Sliced zucchini (2)
- Large grape tomatoes (8)
- Chopped asparagus spears (10)
- Chopped yellow pepper (1)
- Olive oil (2 tbsp.)
- Freshly squeezed lemon juice (1 tbsp.)

- Salt (.5 tsp.)

How To Prepare:

1. Prepare the oven to 450° Fahrenheit. Lightly grease a baking pan.
2. Slice and chop the veggies. Place them into the prepared pan.
3. Toss gently with the oil and juice. Sprinkle with the salt and roast 40 minutes. Stir every 10 minutes to prevent sticking and allow even cooking.

DELICIOUS SNACKS & DESSERTS

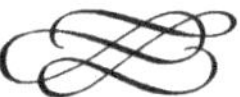

Almond Creamy & Dark Chocolate Bombs

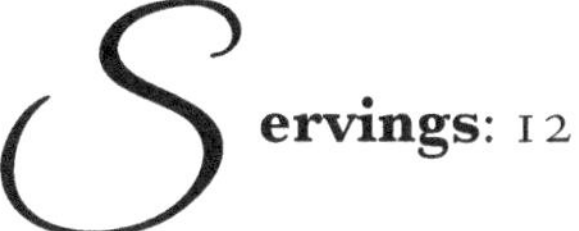

ervings: 12

Total Macro Nutrients:

- 2 g Net Carbs
- 2 g Total Protein
- 7 g Total Fats
- 86 Calories

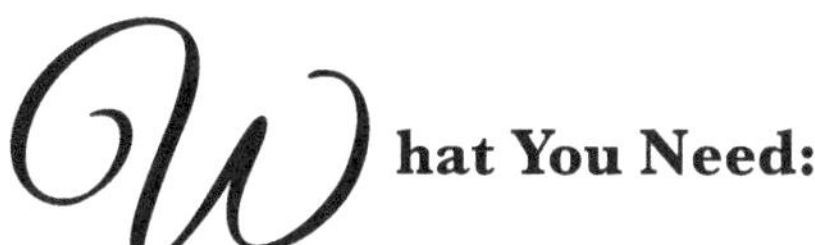

hat You Need:

- Regular cream cheese (1 oz.)
- Coconut butter - not oil (4 tbsp.)
- Almond butter (4 tbsp.)
- 73% organic super dark chocolate - 2 sections
- Sugar-free French vanilla syrup (2 tbsp.)
- Cocoa powder - unsweetened (1 tbsp.)
- Optional: 2 packets of stevia/sweetener of choice

How To Prepare:

1. In a microwavable dish, add all fixings except the coconut butter.
2. Cook at 15-second intervals until the chocolate has melted. Stir all ingredients until incorporated.
3. Spoon the batter into 12 muffin tins or use silicone candy molds.
4. Place the container of bombs in the freezer for about one hour.
5. Just quickly pop them out using a butter knife. Store and enjoy!

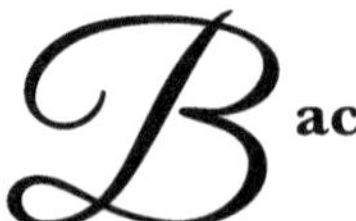

acon Guacamole Fat Bombs

ervings: 6

Total Macro Nutrients:

- 1.4 g Net Carbs
- 3.4 g Total Protein
- 15.2 g Total Fats
- 156 Calories

What You Need

- Avocado (3.5 oz. or about .5 of 1 large)
- Bacon (about 4 oz. - 4 strips)
- Ghee or butter (.25 cup)
- Crushed cloves of garlic (2)
- Small diced onion (approximately 1.2 oz. or .5 of 1)
- Small finely chopped chili pepper (1)
- Fresh lime juice (1 tbsp. or about .25 of a lime)
- Pinch of ground black pepper or cayenne (1 pinch)
- Salt (to your liking)
- Freshly chopped cilantro (1-2 tbsp.)

How To Prepare:

1. Heat up the oven temperature to 375° Fahrenheit. Prepare a baking tray with parchment paper and cook the bacon for 10 to 15 minutes. Save the grease for step four.

2. Peel, deseed, and chop the avocado into a dish along with the garlic, chili pepper, lime juice, cilantro, black pepper, salt, and butter. Use a fork or potato masher to combine the mixture. Blend in the onion.
3. Empty the grease into the bomb fixings, blend well, and cover for 20 to 30 minutes in the fridge.
4. Break up the bacon into a bowl and roll the six balls in it until coated evenly. Serve or eat when you want a delicious snack.

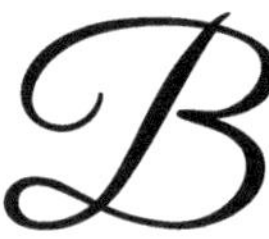

acon Wrapped Mozzarella Sticks

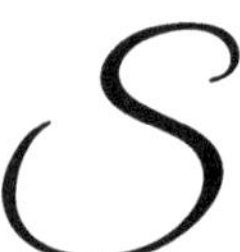

ervings: 2

Total Macro Nutrients:

- 1 g Net Carbs
- 7 g Total Protein
- 9 g Total Fats
- 103 Calories

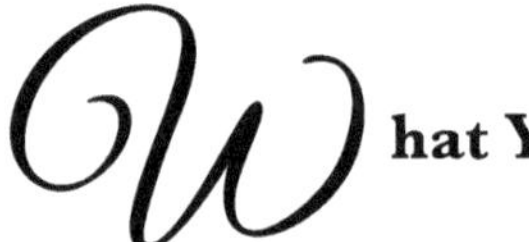

hat You Need:

- Thick bacon (2 slices)
- Frigo cheese head mozzarella cheese sticks (1)
- Coconut oil – for frying

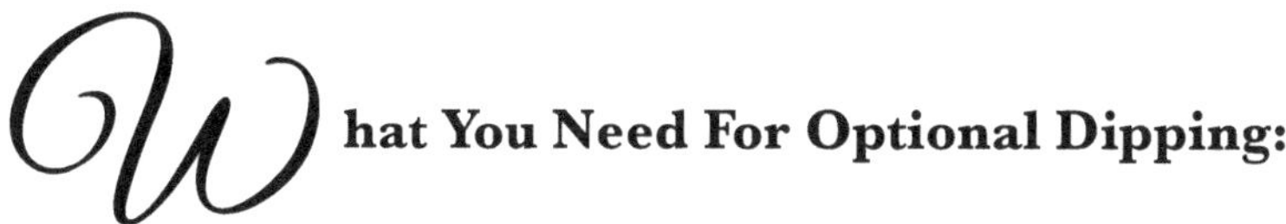

What You Need For Optional Dipping:

- Low-sugar pizza sauce
- Toothpicks

How To Prepare:

1. Warm up the oil to 350° Fahrenheit in a deep fryer.
2. Slice the cheese stick in half. Wrap it with the bacon and secure it closed using the toothpick.
3. Cook the sticks in the hot fryer for 2-3 minutes.
4. Drain on a towel and cool. Serve with your sauce.

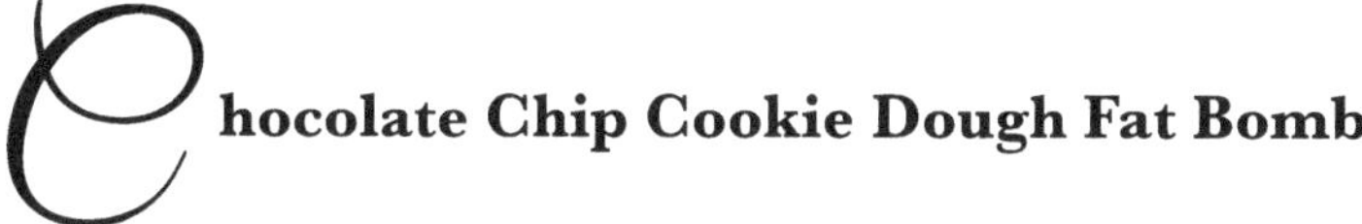

Chocolate Chip Cookie Dough Fat Bomb

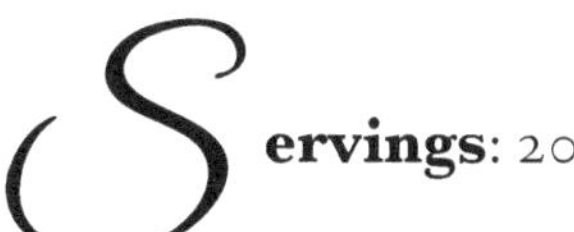

Servings: 20

Total Macro Nutrients:

- 2 g Net Carbs
- 2 g Total Protein
- 14 g Total Fats
- 139 Calories

What You Need:

- Cream cheese (1 pkg. - 8 oz.)
- Salted butter (.5 cup or 1 stick)
- Sweetener – swerve/erythritol (.33 cup)
- Almond butter or creamy peanut butter - only salt and peanuts (.5 cup)
- Vanilla extract (1 tsp.)
- Baking chips - stevia sweetened chocolate chips (4 oz.)

How To Prepare:

1. Remove the cream cheese from the fridge for about 20 to 30 minutes to soften.
2. Use a mixer to blend all of the fixings. Refrigerate at least 30 minutes before adding them onto a tray lined with a layer of parchment paper.
3. Spray an ice cream scoop with a spritz of cooking spray (preferably coconut oil).
4. Scoop out 20 bomb portions and place them onto the prepared pan.
5. Freeze for a minimum of 30 minutes.
6. Store in the fridge in a zipper-type plastic bag for convenience.

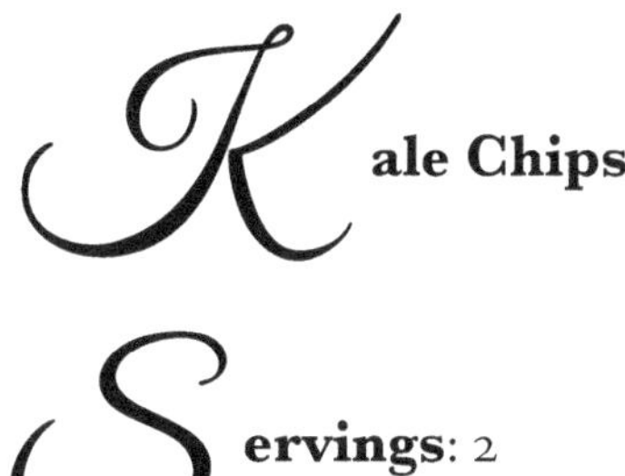

ale Chips

Servings: 2

Total Macro Nutrients:

- 0.5 g Net Carbs
- 4 g Total Protein
- 8 g Total Fats
- 180 Calories

What You Need:

- Kale (1 bunch)
- Crushed red pepper (1 tsp.)
- Garlic powder (1 tsp.)
- Olive oil (2 tbsp.)
- Parmesan cheese (2 tbsp.)

How To Prepare:

1. Program the oven setting until it reaches 350° Fahrenheit.
2. Rinse and dry the kale. Tear it into pieces.

3. Pour the oil over the pieces and toss to combine. Evenly arrange the kale on a baking tin.
4. Bake for 8 minutes. If they are not done, continue baking, checking at 2-minute intervals (approximately 12 min. should be okay).
5. Cool them down for several minutes. Serve when they're crunchy the way you like them.

Desserts

Blackberry Almond Chia Pudding

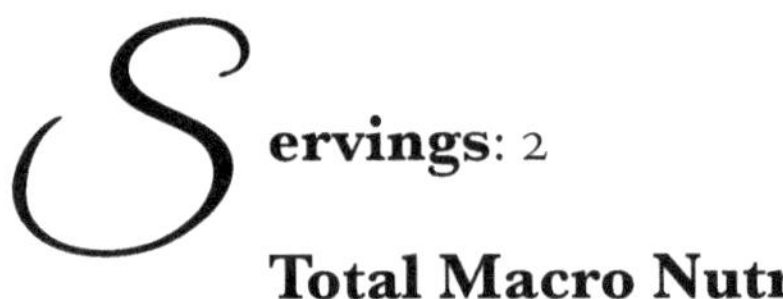

ervings: 2

Total Macro Nutrients:

- 1 g Net Carbs
- 2 g Total Protein
- 8 g Total Fats
- 109 Calories

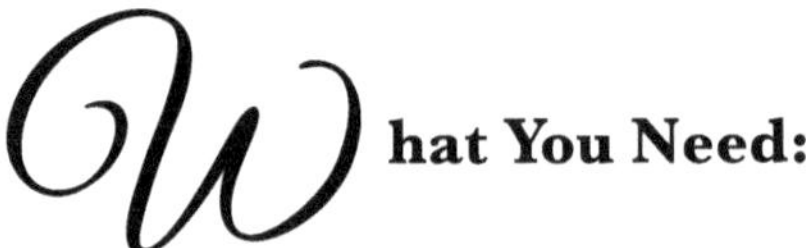

hat You Need:

- Chia seeds (.25 cup)
- Raw honey (drizzle)
- Sliced almonds (2-3 tbsp.)
- Vanilla almond milk (1.5 cups)
- Fresh blackberries (6 oz.)

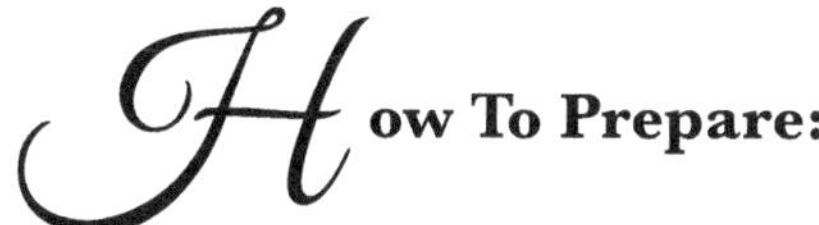

How To Prepare:

1. Rinse and add the berries into a dish. Crush with a fork until creamy.
2. Pour in the raw honey, milk, and chia seeds. Stir well.
3. Refrigerate for several hours or overnight for the most delicious results.
4. Sprinkle with the almonds and several blackberries.
5. Serve any time.

No-Bake Chocolate Peanut Butter Fat Bombs

Servings: 8

Total Macro Nutrients:

- 0.8 g Net Carbs
- 4.4 g Total Protein
- 20 g Total Fats
- 208 Calories

What You Need:

- Shelled hemp seeds (6 tbsp.)

- PB Fit Powder (4 tbsp.)
- Coconut oil (.5 cup)
- Heavy cream (2 tbsp.)
- Cocoa powder (.25 cup)
- Unsweetened shredded coconut (.25 cup)
- Liquid stevia (28 drops)
- Vanilla extract (1 tsp.)

How To Prepare:

1. Combine all of the dry fixings and blend in the oil which will create a paste.
2. Mix the heavy cream, stevia, and vanilla into the paste - until just combined. Shape into eight balls.
3. Dump the coconut on a flat surface. Roll the balls through it.
4. Arrange the balls in a dish. Store in the freezer compartment for a minimum of 20 minutes.

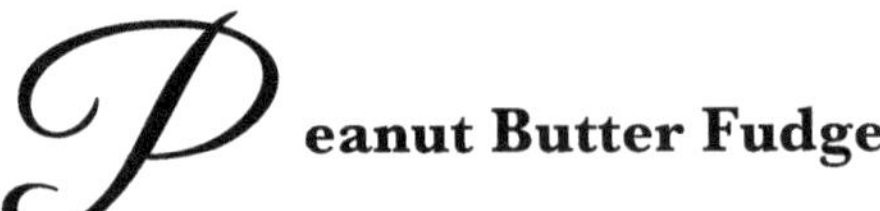

Peanut Butter Fudge

Servings: 18

Total Macro Nutrients:

- -0- g Net Carbs
- 2 g Total Protein

- 8 g Total Fats
- 89 Calories

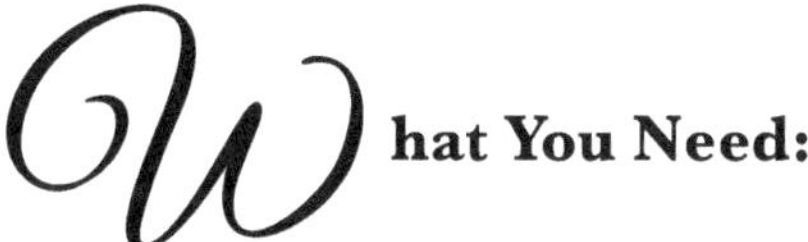

What You Need:

- Coconut oil (.5 cup)
- Peanut butter (.5 cup)
- Liquid stevia granulated sweetener (as desired)
- Also Needed: 12-18 count muffin tin & liners or a loaf pan

How To Prepare:

1. Prepare the tin of choice with a spritz of oil.
2. Combine the oil and peanut butter together on the stovetop or microwave. Melt and add the sweetener.
3. Scoop into the tins or loaf pan and freeze.
4. You can serve with a drizzle of melted chocolate – but remember to count the carbs.

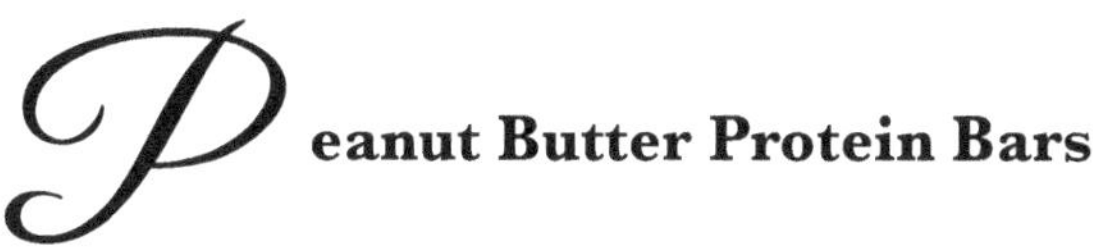

Peanut Butter Protein Bars

. . .

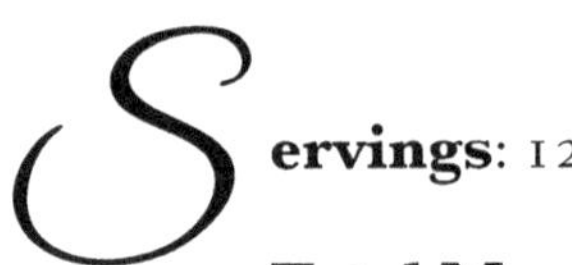

Servings: 12

Total Macro Nutrients:

- 3 g Net Carbs
- 7 g Total Protein
- 14 g Total Fats
- 172 Calories

What You Need:

- Almond meal (1.5 cups)
- Keto-friendly chunky peanut butter (1 cup)
- Egg whites (2)
- Almonds (.5 cup)
- Cashews (.5 cup)
- Also Needed: Baking pan

How To Prepare:

1. Heat the oven ahead of time to reach 350° Fahrenheit.
2. Spritz a baking dish lightly with coconut or olive oil.
3. Combine all of the fixings and add to the prepared dish.
4. Bake for 15 minutes and cut into 12 pieces once they're cooled.

5. Store in the refrigerator to keep them fresh.

Pumpkin Bread

ervings: 8

Total Macro Nutrients:

- 5 g Net Carbs
- 8 g Total Protein
- 26 g Total Fats
- 311 Calories

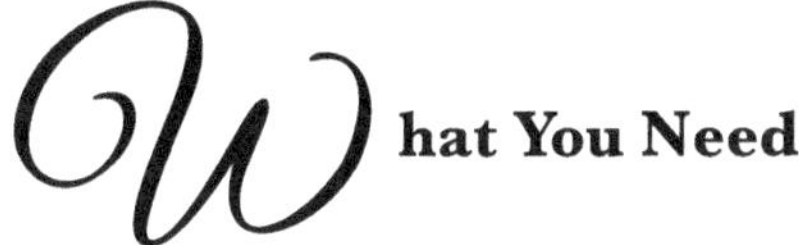

hat You Need

- Almond flour (1 cup)
- Libby's Canned Pumpkin (1 small can)
- Baking powder (.5 tsp.)
- Coconut flour (.5 cup)
- Heavy cream (.5 cup)
- Stevia (.5 cup)
- Melted butter (1 stick)
- Large eggs (4)
- Vanilla (1.5 tsp.)
- Pumpkin spice (2 tsp.)

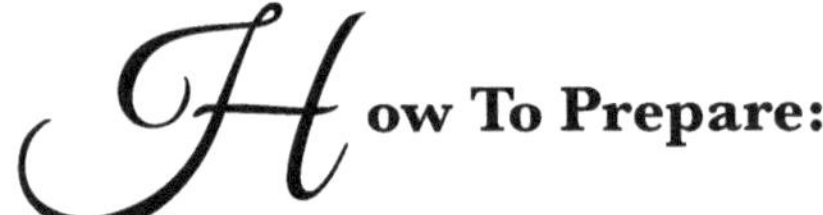

How To Prepare:

1. Set the oven temperature setting to 350° Fahrenheit. Grease a pie plate with a spritz of coconut oil.
2. Combine all of the fixings in a mixing container until light and fluffy.
3. Pour the batter into the prepared pan. Bake for approximately 70 to 90 minutes.

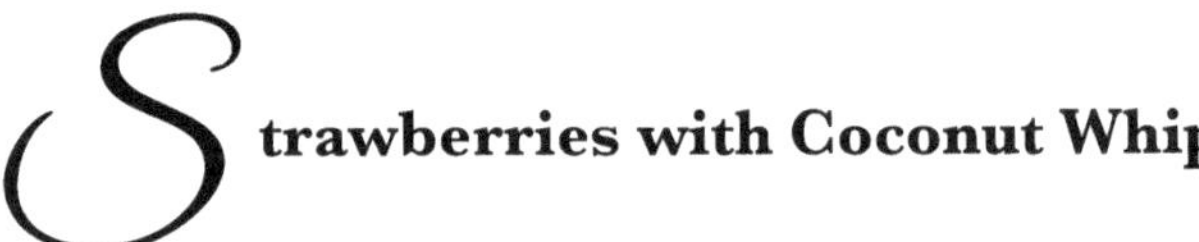

Strawberries with Coconut Whip

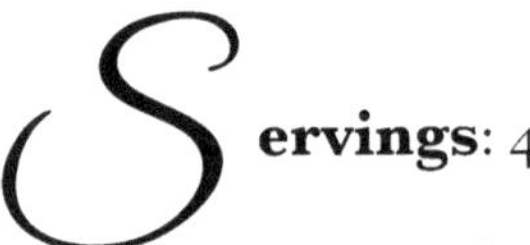

Servings: 4

Total Macro Nutrients:

- 10 g Net Carbs
- 4 g Total Protein
- 31 g Total Fats
- 342 Calories

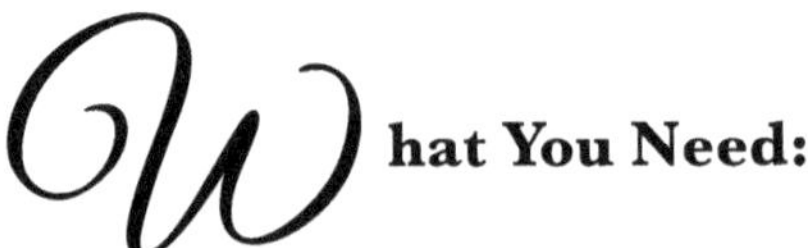

What You Need:

- Strawberries or other favorite berries (4 cups)
- Refrigerated coconut cream (2 cans)

- Unsweetened chopped dark chocolate - 70% or darker (1 oz.)

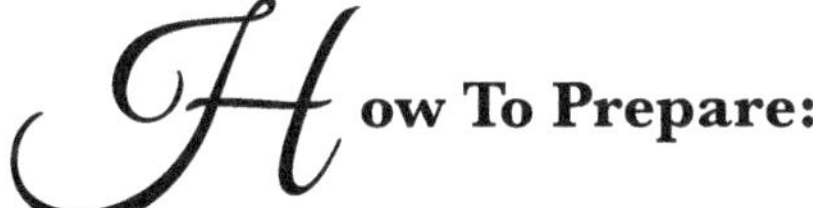

How To Prepare:

1. Remove the solidified cream from the can of milk and set aside for another time, saving the liquid. Pour it into a mixing container and whip with a hand mixer until it forms stiff peaks (approximately five minutes).
2. Slice the berries and portion into four dishes. Serve with a dollop of the cream. Garnish with the chopped chocolate and a few berries. Serve.

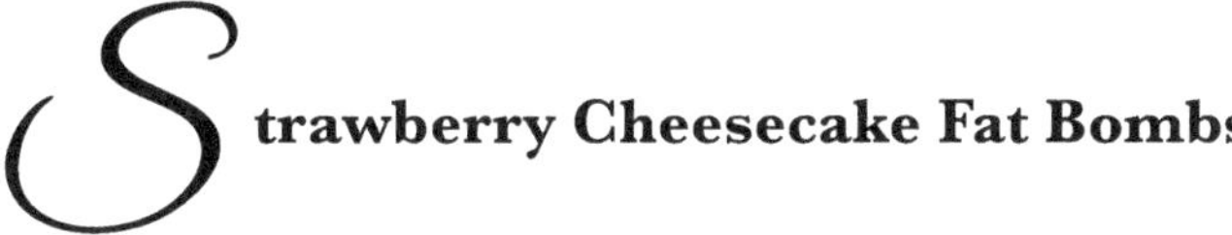

Strawberry Cheesecake Fat Bombs

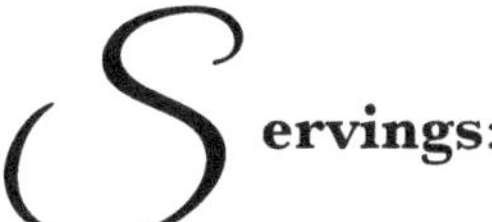

Servings: 12

Total Macro Nutrients:

- 0.85 g Net Carbs
- 0.96 g Total Protein
- 7.4 g Total Fats
- 67 Calories

What You Need:

- Coconut oil or softened butter (.25 cup)
- Softened cream cheese (.75 cup)
- Fresh/frozen strawberries (.5 cup)
- Liquid stevia (10-15 drops) or powdered erythritol (2 tbsp.)
- Vanilla extract (1 tbsp.)

How To Prepare:

1. Mix the butter or coconut oil with the cream cheese in a mixing container. Let it rest 30-60 minutes until it is room temperature. (Don't microwave.)
2. Prepare the berries and remove the stems. Add them to a dish and mash until smooth. Stir in the stevia and vanilla. Mix well using a food processor or hand whisk.
3. Scoop out the mixture and add into candy molds or muffin silicone molds.
4. Let the bombs rest in the freezer until set, usually about two hours.
5. Just pop them out and enjoy. Store in the freezer.

Strawberry Thumbprint Delights

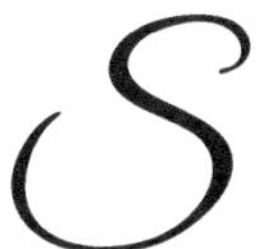

Servings: 16

Total Macro Nutrients:

- 1 g Net Carbs
- 2 g Total Protein
- 9 g Total Fats
- 95 Calories

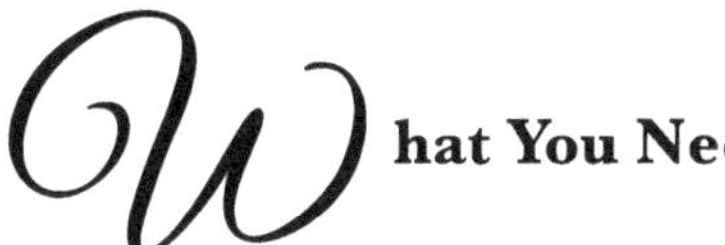

What You Need:

- Almond flour (1 cup)
- Baking powder (.5 tsp.)
- Coconut flour (2 tbsp.)
- Sugar-free strawberry jam (2 tbsp.)
- Shredded coconut (1 tbsp.)
- Eggs (2)
- Erythritol (.5 cup)
- Coconut oil (4 tbsp.)
- Salt (.5 tsp.)
- Cinnamon (.5 tsp.)
- Almond extract (.5 tsp.)
- Vanilla extract (.5 tsp.)

How To Prepare:

1. Warm up the oven temperature to 350° Fahrenheit. Cover a cookie tin with a sheet of parchment paper.
2. Whisk the dry fixings and make a hole in the middle. Fold in the wet fixings to form a dough. Break it into 16 segments and roll into balls.
3. Arrange each one on the prepared cookie sheet and bake 15 minutes.
4. When done, cool completely and add a dab of jam to each one with a sprinkle of coconut.

CONCLUSION

I sincerely hope that you enjoyed each segment of the *Intermittent Fasting: A Guide to Burn Fat, Weight Loss, Improve Health, Healing – Low Carb Keto Diet Recipes.* I hope it was informative and provided you with all of the tools you need to achieve your goals of losing weight and to become healthier. As you read through your new book, many simple tips were provided for your ketogenic journey. These are just several of them, so you have them fresh in your mind:

- Drink plenty of water daily and limit the intake of sugar-sweetened beverages.
- Use only fat-free or low-fat condiments.
- Read the food labels and make choices that keep you in line with ketosis.
- Add a serving of vegetables to your dinner and lunch menus.
- For a snack, have some frozen yogurt (fat-free or low-fat),

nuts or unsalted pretzels, raw veggies, or unsalted-plain popcorn.

One last recipe for success:

Bone Broth

This remedy has been around for many years. The broth can eliminate keto flu symptoms and provide you with an increase of your essential electrolytes. The broth can boost your immune system, help keep your intestinal tract healthier, and increase collagen levels to improve your eyes, heart, skin, joints, and bones. You will also achieve improved brain health.

Make yourself a batch anytime to sip or use in your cooking. Use the recipe below:

Servings: 6-8 cups

Total Macro Nutrients:

- 0.7 g Net Carbs
- 3.6 g Total Protein
- 6 g Total Fats
- 72 Calories

What You Need

- Mixed assorted bones – ex. marrow bones, chicken feet, pork or your choice (3.5 lb.)
- Pink Himalayan salt (1 tbsp.)
- Medium parsnip (1)
- Medium white onion – skin on (1)
- Minced garlic (5 cloves)

- Medium celery (2 stalks)
- Medium Carrots (2)
- Apple cider vinegar or lemon juice (2 tbsp.)
- Water (8 cups)
- Also Needed: Slow cooker

How To Prepare:

1. Peel and slice the vegetables with roots into 1/3-inch pieces. Slice the onion in half. Chop the celery into thirds. Add the bay leaves into the slow cooker.
2. Toss in the chosen bones. Pour the water up to ¾ capacity – along with the juice/vinegar, and bay leaves. Sprinkle with the salt.
3. Secure the lid. Choose either low (ten hours) or high (six hours). You can simmer up to 48 hours.
4. Use a strainer to remove the bits of veggies. Set the bones aside to chill. Shred the meat and use as desired.
5. Refrigerate the broth overnight. Scrape away the tallow (greasy layer) if desired. Use within five days or freeze. You can also keep it in the canning jars for up to 45 days.

By now, you have decided which of the intermittent fasting techniques you will be using on this journey. Try one of the plans and give it some time for your body to adjust. This is not a miracle diet but a new way of living. You also know how you can best mix and match to find the perfect solution for you. Making the decision to alter your original eating patterns is a major one, and it is crucial that you take the full weight of the decision into account before acting.

If you are convinced that you have what it takes to take full advantage of the benefits that intermittent fasting has to offer, then the next step is to stop reading and to start fasting. Choose the type of intermittent fasting technique that seems like the best fit for you and give it a try. You have a plentiful supply of recipes to use to begin the program.

Try not to become discouraged if you don't receive immediate results. Make an effort to find the one that's right for you. Above all, don't rush, and remember, intermittent fasting is a marathon not a sprint, slow and steady will win the race.

Finally, if you found this book useful in any way, a review on Amazon is always appreciated!

INDEX

Smoothies

CPSIA information can be obtained
at www.ICGtesting.com
Printed in the USA
LVHW080035030521
686310LV00013B/702